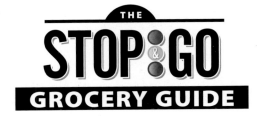

THE STOP & GO GROCERY GUIDE

By Steven G. Aldana, PhD

with Monique Hess, MS

The Stop & Go Grocery Guide

Wellness Council of America
9802 Nicholas Street, Suite 315
Omaha, NE 68114
phone: (402) 827-3590
email: wellworkplace@welcoa.org

ISBN: 978-097588289-4

Printed in the United States of America

Layout design and art direction by Brad Moulton
Maple Mountain Studio | www.maplemountainstudio.com

Table of Contents

Introduction

Food Categories

You are a caveman. At least your body still thinks so. The human body is pretty darn similar to the bodies of the earliest humans. Culturally and socially, we exist in a rapidly changing 21st century, but our bodies have not changed much compared to the bodies of earliest humans.[1] The truth is, we are all Paleolithic.

As a species, humans have been around for a very long time.[2] For nearly all of human history, our ancestors lived off the land. They hunted wild game and gathered fruits, vegetables and roots. As they ate what was available to them, their bodies adapted. For example, their stomachs got used to digesting whole, natural foods like onions, apples, and wild rice; their cells became accustomed to being bathed in plant-based chemicals; and their teeth adapted to better grind and chew food. Our bodies inherited these abilities from those who preceded us. We have been prepared since time began to hunt, gather, and eat wholesome food just like our ancient ancestors. But we no longer share the same diet. Cavemen did not consume Hostess Twinkies™, Kellogg's Sugar Frosted Flakes™, or diet Dr. Pepper™. We've changed.

White sugar has only been part of our diet for about 200 years. White flour has only been publicly available for about 150 years. The most widely consumed sweetener, high-fructose corn syrup, has only been around for about 45 years.[3-5] White sugar, white flour and, high-fructose cornsyrup are dietary newbies. In fact, if all of human history were contained in a single day, then white flour would have been part of our diet for about two minutes.

What you see in stores today are modern foods. Most did not exist 100 years ago. It is hard to imagine that 99.9 percent of all humans ever born never tasted Reese's Puffs™ Breakfast Cereal.

The foods largely available today resulted from the industrial revolution and our free market system. Modern food is abundant, inexpensive and not as compatible with our ancient bodies. Early humans did not eat cheese, butter, sugars, syrups, refined flours, vegetable oils, shortening, margarine or added salt.[6] They did eat meat, but not the kind we eat. Today, 99% of all beef is produced from grain-fed, feedlot cattle. This meat is not as healthy as meat that comes from animals that have been allowed to free range.[7]

It is true that ancient humans suffered from many illnesses and diseases that we no longer experience. They worked hard and typically died young. Yet, despite these health challenges, it appears that they did not have type II diabetes, heart disease, obesity, and other now-common chronic diseases.[8] This is why I wrote this guide:

Most of the chronic diseases that afflict the industrial world are caused by a diet and lifestyle that is inconsistent with the ancient bodies we inherited from our ancestors.

Still Not Convinced?

Here is what we know from the best available science. Many scientists from around the world have tried to identify the ideal diet by studying the relationship between the foods people eat and the diseases they get later in life. After decades of research on thousands and thousands of people, they have identified two dietary patterns that either cause or prevent chronic diseases. The diet that is the most unhealthy has been called "The Western diet." People that eat a Western diet typically live in industrialized countries that are "Westernized" or more like America—and not in a good way! This Western diet includes lots of red meat, french fries, refined flours, butter, processed meats, high-fat dairy products, sweets, desserts, few fruits, and even fewer vegetables.

The dietary pattern that is associated with good health is called "The Prudent diet." The Prudent diet contains mostly whole grains, plant oils, vegetables, fruits, and legumes as illustrated in the pyramid below.

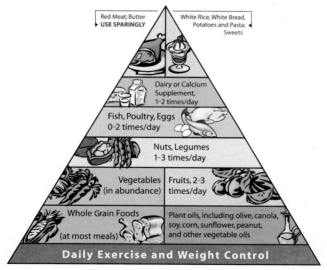

Healthy Eating Pyramid

The Prudent Diet Pattern
http://www.hsph.harvard.edu/nutritionsource
[ ] th permission.

The foods on the bottom of the pyramid should be the primary source of energy. The foods on the top of the pyramid should be eaten sparingly. The Prudent diet is based on whole foods that are either in or very close to their natural state. These are foods that would have been part of any human diet since day one. Interestingly, if the pyramid were flipped upside down it would very accurately depict the Western diet.

What happens to those who follow the Prudent diet and the Western diet? Through large studies with hundreds of thousands of participants, researchers have determined important differences between those who follow both diets. Those who follow the Prudent diet lower their risk of diabetes by 16% and heart disease by 34%. By contrast, those who eat a Western diet increase their risk of diabetes by 59%,[9-10] and heart disease by 64%.[11-13] These two diet patterns are associated in the same way with other chronic diseases such as colon cancer,[14] stroke,[15] Parkinson's Disease, breast cancer, stomach cancer, asthma, and obesity.[16-20] Bottom line? Eat like a caveman (a Prudent diet) to reduce your risk of chronic disease.

The research is clear. Eating whole foods is the best way to maintain a healthy weight and avoid chronic diseases.

How this Guide Will Help You Eat like a Caveman.

To have really good health and avoid most chronic diseases, you should eat whole foods—foods that are in or close to their natural form. For example, fresh produce is whole food. It is in it's natural form. It was grown, cleaned, packed, and sent to the store or market for purchase. Produce is an example of a basic whole food that humans have been eating for thousands of years. They are easy to identify and everyone knows they are good for you. But what about all the other foods in the grocery store? How can you tell if a food is close to its natural form? Take Quaker™ oatmeal for example. Quaker Old Fashion Oatmeal is a pretty basic food. It is not quite in its natural form, but it is close. Most oatmeal we purchase has been processed with a big roller that flattens the oat kernels. It is still an oat kernel, just flat. Quaker Old Fashion Oatmeal is an example of a grocery store food that is close to its original form and is good for you.

What about Quaker Dinosaur Eggs Brown Sugar Oatmeal? Do you think this is really a whole food? If you said, "No," you were correct. Oatmeal is listed as an ingredient alright, but it is not even close to it's natural form. It has been processed until it is unrecognizable. But kids still love it because it has a cool name.

The word "processed" refers to all the changes that food can undergo before it actually ends up on your plate. Some of this processing is actually good. Foods can be sterilized, pasteurized, chopped up, dehydrated, or frozen. These processes can make food safer and more nutritious.

But there is a dark side to food processing. Let's talk about oatmeal again. Do you remember Lucky Charms™ breakfast cereal? Lucky Charms cereal is made from oats, but you wouldn't know it unless you carefully examined the ingredients. General Mills, the manufacturer of Lucky Charms, calls them a whole grain, frosted oats cereal and boasts that they are "magically delicious."

Here are the ingredients of Lucky Charms:
Oat flour, marshmallow bits (sugar, modified corn starch, corn syrup, dextrose, gelatin, calcium carbonate, yellow 5&6, blue 1, red 40, artificial flavor), sugar, corn syrup, corn starch, salt, calcium carbonate, color added, trisodium phosphate, zinc and iron (mineral nutrients), vitamin C (sodium ascorbate), a B vitamin (niacinamide), artificial flavor, vitamin B6 (pyridoxine hydrochloride), vitamin B2 (riboflavin), vitamin B1 (thiamin mononitrate), vitamin A (palmitate), a B vitamin (folic acid), vitamin B12, vitamin D, wheat starch, vitamin E (mixed tocopherols) added to preserve freshness.

Even though the few oats that are in Lucky Charms are actually whole oats (the shell, germ, and starch of the oat kernel), this cereal is far from being a whole food. Even worse, it presents a real challenge to our ancient physiology and our overall good health.

Can you imagine what the early cavemen would do if they found a box of Lucky Charms cereal with colorful marshmallow bits? Lucky Charms is a good example of a food that has undergone so much processing that it can no longer be considered a food that contributes to good health. General Mills Lucky Charms are coded "red" in this guide as a warning that they should be avoided or eaten very sparingly. The truth is, eating a box of Lucky Charms cereal will not kill you. But if most of your diet consists of processed foods like Lucky Charms, your risk of getting a chronic disease is probably higher.

Let's be honest. It is really hard to choose foods that are healthy. Food producers know this and are not interested in helping you make healthy choices. They are more interested in profits than they are in your health. In fact, they have a financial motive to sell as much food as possible. To do so, they will try to convince you that their processed foods are healthy by using marketing tactics that are deceptive at best and big fat lies at worst. Don't be fooled.

It's All About the Money

Are you still reading this? If so, I must have your full attention. Would you like to know what I really think? Here it is. I have spent most of my adult life trying to help people live a more healthy life. I have spent a lot of time thinking about why it is so hard to eat healthy foods and I've come to a few conclusions. Here is one: We eat unhealthy foods because we are easily fooled by the marketing efforts and messages of food producers.

Food producers want to make money. Period. Take a look at a box of Cocoa Puffs™ Cereal. Look on the side panel and you'll see the heart shaped label of the American Heart Association (AHA). This American Heart Association label means that the food manufacturer has met some sort of nutrition recommendation. It also means that the food manufacturer has given the AHA thousands of dollars. In essence, the food producers have purchased the blessing of the AHA. The food producers will sell more product with the official blessing of the AHA and the AHA makes millions of dollars each year in labeling fees. This situation is a win-win,–lose. The food producers win. The AHA wins. The consumer loses.

The nutrition labeling approach to food marketing is a common practice and it is a big business. Remember, it's all about the money. Food producers know that you will make purchasing decisions based on these labels. For example, the Whole Grain Council came up with some simple food rules for a Whole Grain Stamp. Any food producer that meets the rules and pays their fee, $1,000–$10,000 per year, gets the right to use the Whole Grain Stamp. Some foods that carry this stamp are actually healthy but many are not. Pepsico™ thumbed its nose at all the other labels and started their own called Smart Spot. Over 250 Pepsico™ products now carry the Smart Spot label. Some of the nation's biggest food producers, General Mills, Kellogg, Kraft Foods, and others got together and created their own label called Smart Choices.

The foods you see in grocery stores are now plastered with these self-serving labels and stamps. It is the food producer equivalent of "keeping up with the Jones." Each is trying to beat the competition with bigger and bolder health claims and labels. But what do the claims really mean? They mean that the consumer will buy more. They mean that you will often pay more. But they do not mean you will be healthier. In fact, eating cleverly disguised unhealthy food will lead to just as much weight gain, chronic disease, and premature death as obviously unhealthy food like donuts. Nobody would dare slap a healthy label on a donut would they?

How this Guide Can Help

The purpose of this guide is to help you purchase and eat more whole foods. There are over 300,000 different foods that can be purchased in grocery stores. It was simply impossible to include all of them in this guide. To keep this guide at a manageable size, it has been limited to the top selling 3,500 foods in the U.S. The nutrition information for each food was then added into a food database. Finally, each of these foods was placed into one of 14 food categories. These categories are the same ones grocery stores use to organize and display foods. The categories include:

Baked Goods & Doughs	Condiments & Sauces	Packaged Dinners
Baking Items	Dairy	Pasta and Rice
Beverages	Frozen Foods	Produce
Breakfast Foods	Meats	Snacks
Canned Goods	Packaged Desserts	

To find a food, go to the category in which the food is normally found. The foods are listed alphabetically by brand within each category. If you can't find your food, look in the index at the end of the book to make sure you are looking in the right category. If you still can't find your food, it is possible the food is not in the guide. In this case, just use the five simple rules suggested by Michael Pollan in his book, "In Defense of Food: An Eater's Manifesto."

1. Don't eat anything your great grandmother wouldn't recognize as food. (Or don't eat anything that doesn't rot).

2. Avoid food products containing ingredients that are a) unfamiliar, b) unpronounceable, c) more than five in number, or include d) high-fructose corn syrup.

3. Avoid food products that make health claims.

4. Shop the peripheries of the supermarket and stay out of the middle.

5. Get out of the supermarket whenever possible—shake the hand that feeds you.

I like these rules, they can help you choose well when the guide does not.

Just Follow the Colors

With the assistance of a team of nutrition experts, a set of rules and guidelines was created to classify foods according to nutritional value. These classifications are based on the nutrition information from each food. There is nothing magical about these rules except that they give some indication as to whether or not a food is close to, or far from, its original form. From these rules, a red, yellow and green color coding process was developed.

Because of space constraints, there was a limit to the amount of nutrition information that could be included in this guide. **It is important to note that the color coding is based on much more than just the nutrition information shown in the guide.**

There is an easier way to think about the color coding rules. By using the Prudent diet pyramid discussed earlier, foods can be coded according to where they are located on the pyramid. Healthy green-coded foods would be those on the bottom of the pyramid; yellow towards the middle; and red foods, which should be eaten sparingly, located on the top.

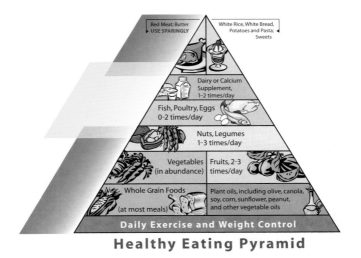

Healthy Eating Pyramid

The red, yellow, and green color coding system is simple. Anyone can use the guide to make healthier choices. Here are three easy rules to help you use this system to make healthy food choices:

Rule #1: Avoid the red foods.

Rule #2: Go easy on the yellow foods.

Rule #3: Eat healthy with the green foods.

Red foods = Hit the brakes!

Foods that are colored red earn this color because they are considered to be the least healthy within a food category. They may contain a lot of sodium, trans fats, saturated fat, refined flour, sugars, or a lot of additional processing. Just over 60% of the foods in this guide are colored red. That's because a majority of the most popular grocery store foods are not very healthy.

Yellow foods = Exercise caution!

Foods that are coded yellow are better than the red ones, but fall short of being considered a green food. About 20% of the foods in this guide are coded yellow.

Green foods = You're eatin' healthy!

Green foods are the best and should be the primary source of dietary intake. Obviously fresh produce, nuts, seeds, and whole grains are coded green, but so are foods made with substantial whole grains, fruits, vegetables, and healthy oils. Green-coded foods include vegetable pizza, many frozen foods, canned foods, and prepared dinners with ample whole foods such as vegetable stir-fry. Green foods are low in saturated and trans fats, they don't contain excessive amounts of sodium or cholesterol, and they are relatively low in calories compared to yellow and red foods. They are actually good for you and should be eaten every day.

In this guide all of the best-selling foods are color coded. With the color coding it is possible to identify the best and worst food brands. Here are the top-ten best and worst brands.

Top 10 brands with the most green foods:

Barilla	Green Giant
Bird's Eye	Hunt's
Dannon	Minute Maid/Tropicana (similar)
Del Monte	Progresso
Dole	Ragu

Top 10 brands with the most red foods:

Betty Crocker	Kellogg's
Campbell's	Kraft
Dreyer's/Edy's	Nabisco
Entenmann's	Pillsbury
General Mills	Stouffer's

REFERENCES

1. Cordain L, Eaton SB, Sebastian A, Mann N, Lindeberg S, Watkins BA, O'Keefe JH, Brand-Miller J. *Origins and evolution of the Western diet: health implications for the 21st century.* Am J Clin Nutr. 2005 Feb;81(2):341-54.

2. Wood B. Hominid revelations from Chad. *Nature.* 2002 Jul 11;418(6894):133-5.

3. Storck J. Teague WD. *Flour for Man's Bread, a history of milling.* Minneapolis: University of Minnesota Press, 1952

4. Galloway JH. 2000. *Sugar.* In: Kiple KF, Ornelas IKC, eds. *The Cambridge world history of food. Vol 1.* Cambridge: Cambridge University Press, 2000:437-49.

5. Hanover LM, White JS. *Manufacturing, composition, and applications of fructose.* Am J Clin Nutr. 1993 Nov;58(5 Suppl):724S-732S.

6. Gerrior S, Bente L. *Nutrient content of the U.S. food supply, 1909-1999: a summary report.* Washington, DC: US Department of Agriculture, Center for Nutrition Policy and Promotion, 2002.

7. Kidwell B. *All grass, no grain. Progressive Farmer Magazine,* 8 October 2002.

8. O'Keefe JH Jr, Cordain L. *Cardiovascular disease resulting from a diet and lifestyle at odds with our Paleolithic genome: how to become a 21st-century hunter-gatherer.* Mayo Clin Proc. 2004 Jan;79(1):101-8.

9. van Dam RM, Rimm EB, Willett WC, Stampfer MJ, Hu FB. *Dietary patterns and risk for type 2 diabetes mellitus in U.S. men.* Ann Intern Med. 2002 Feb 5;136(3):201–9.

10. Hu FB, Manson JE, Stampfer MJ, Colditz G, Liu S, Solomon CG, Willett WC. *Diet, lifestyle, and the risk of type 2 diabetes mellitus in women.* N Engl J Med. 2001 Sep 13;345(11):790–7.

11. Fung TT, Willett WC, Stampfer MJ, Manson JE, Hu FB. *Dietary patterns and the risk of coronary heart disease in women.* Arch Intern Med. 2001 Aug 13-27;161(15):1857–62.

12. Schulze MB, Hu FB. *Dietary patterns and risk of hypertension, type 2 diabetes mellitus, and coronary heart disease.* Curr Atheroscler Rep. 2002 Nov;4(6):462–7.

13. Millen BE, Quatromoni PA, Nam BH, O'Horo CE, Polak JF, Wolf PA, D'Agostino RB; *Framingham Nutrition Studies. Dietary patterns, smoking, and subclinical heart disease in women: opportunities for primary prevention from the Framingham Nutrition Studies.* J Am Diet Assoc. 2004 Feb;104(2):208-14.

14. Terry P, Hu FB, Hansen H, Wolk A. *Prospective study of major dietary patterns and colorectal cancer risk in women.* Am J Epidemiol. 2001 Dec 15;154(12):1143–9.

15. Ding EL, Mozaffarian D. *Optimal dietary habits for the prevention of stroke.* Semin Neurol. 2006 Feb;26(1):11-23.

16. Agurs-Collins T, Rosenberg L, Makambi K, Palmer JR, Adams-Campbell L. *Dietary patterns and breast cancer risk in women participating in the Black Women's Health Study.* Am J Clin Nutr. 2009 Sep;90(3):621-8.

17. Kwan ML, Weltzien E, Kushi LH, Castillo A, Slattery ML, Caan BJ. *Dietary patterns and breast cancer recurrence and survival among women with early- stage breast cancer.* J Clin Oncol. 2009 Feb 20;27(6):919-26.

18. Varraso R, Kauffmann F, Leynaert B, Le Moual N, Boutron-Ruault MC, Clavel-Chapelon F, Romieu I. *Dietary patterns and asthma in the E3N study.* Eur Respir J. 2009 Jan;33(1):33-41.

19. Gao X, Chen H, Fung TT, Logroscino G, Schwarzschild MA, Hu FB, Ascherio A. *Prospective study of dietary pattern and risk of Parkinson disease.* Am J Clin Nutr. 2007 Nov;86(5):1486-94

20. Murtaugh MA, Herrick JS, Sweeney C, Baumgartner KB, Guiliano AR, Byers T, Slattery ML. *Diet composition and risk of overweight and obesity in women living in the southwestern United States.* J Am Diet Assoc. 2007 Aug;107(8):1311-21.

Baked Goods & Doughs

	Serving	Calories	Total fat (gm)	Saturated fat (gm)	Trans fats (gm)	Cholesterol (mg)	Sodium (mg)	Carbs (gm)
Anzio & Son's White Kaiser Rolls	57g	170	2.5	0.5	0	0	310	31
Arnold 100% Whole Wheat Bread	43g	110	1	0	0	0	220	20
Arnold 12 Grain Bread	38g	110	2	0	0	0	190	19
Arnold 7 Grain Bread	38g	100	1	0	0	0	180	20
Arnold Country Wheat Bread	38g	100	1.5	0	0	0	190	19
Arnold Country White Bread	38g	110	1.5	0	0	0	230	20
Arnold Honey Almond Bread	38g	110	2	0	0	0	190	18
Arnold Italian Bread	30g	80	1	0	0	0	230	15
Arnold Jewish Rye Bread	30g	80	1.5	0	0	0	220	15
Arnold Multigrain Bread	38g	100	1.5	0	0	0	140	18
Arnold Natural Flax & Fiber Bread	33g	80	1.5	0	0	0	160	16
Arnold Natural Health Nut Bread	33g	100	2	0	0	0	160	16
Arnold Oat Bran Bread	38g	100	1	0	0	0	190	18
Arnold Oat Nut Bread	43g	120	2	0	0	0	230	22
Arnold Select 100% Whole Wheat Sandwich Buns	43g	100	1	0	0	0	230	21
Arnold Select Multigrain Sandwich Buns	43g	100	1	0	0	0	230	22
Arnold Select Sesame Sandwich Rolls	50g	150	2.5	0.5	0	0	300	26
Arnold Select Wheat Sandwich Rolls	57g	150	2	0.5	0	0	310	29
Arnold Select White Hamburger Buns	57g	150	2	0.5	0	0	350	30
Arnold White Hot Dog Buns	50g	140	2	0	0	0	290	26
Arnold Grains & More 100% Whole Wheat Bread	43g	100	1.5	0	0	0	200	21
Arnold Grains & More Multigrain Bread	43g	110	2	0	0	0	200	18
Aunt Millie's 100% Whole Wheat Bread	34g	80	1	0	0	0	170	15
Aunt Millie's Country Buttermilk Bread	34g	90	1	0	0	0	160	16
Aunt Millie's Cracked Wheat Bread	34g	80	1	0	0	0	160	15
Azteca Flour Tortillas	48g	130	3	0.5	0	0	390	23
Ball Park White Hot Dog Buns	43g	120	1.5	0	0	0	230	23
Beefsteak Rye Bread	25g	60	0.5	0	0	0	130	12
Bimbo Weight Watchers 100% Whole Wheat Bread	41g	90	1.0	0	0	0	180	17
Bimbo Weight Watchers English Muffins	57g	100	0.5	0	0	0	230	24
Bimbo Weight Watchers Multigrain Bread	41g	100	1.0	0	0	0	170	18
Bimbo Weight Watchers Original Bagels	71g	150	1	0	0	0	350	34
Brownberry 100% Whole Wheat Bread	43g	110	1	0	0	0	210	20
Brownberry 12 Grain Bread	43g	110	2	0	0	0	200	21
Brownberry Country Buttermilk Bread	43g	120	1.5	0.5	0	0	220	22
Brownberry Dutch Country 100% Whole Wheat Bread	38g	90	1	0	0	0	190	18
Brownberry Dutch Country Potato Bread	35g	100	1.5	0	0	0	170	18

Baked Goods & Doughs

	Serving	Calories	Total fat (gm)	Saturated fat (gm)	Trans fats (gm)	Cholesterol (mg)	Sodium (mg)	Carbs (gm)
Brownberry Health Nut Bread	43g	120	2	0	0	0	220	21
Brownberry Oat Nut Bread	43g	120	2.5	0	0	0	240	22
Brownberry Whole Grain Wheat Bread	36g	100	1.5	0	0	0	240	18
Butternut White Bread	26g	60	0.5	0	0	0	130	13
California Goldminer Sourdough Bread	57g	130	0.5	0	0	0	280	26
Cinnabon Cinnamon Bread	38g	120	3	1	0	5	160	20
Country Hearth 12 Grain Bread	34g	90	1.5	0	0	0	160	18
Country Hearth Wheat Bread	28g	70	1	0	0	0	150	14
Country Kitchen Canadian White Bread	39g	110	2.0	0	0	0	260	20
Country Kitchen Wheat Bread	28g	80	1.0	0	0	0	170	16
Country Kitchen White Bread	26g	70	1	0	0	0	135	13
D'Italiano Italian Bread	27g	80	0.5	0	0	0	160	15
Drake's Coffee Cake	65g	260	10	4.5	0	10	170	42
Entenmann's All Butter Pound Cake	57g	220	9	5	0	70	270	30
Entenmann's Chocolate Frosted Devil's Food Donuts	67g	310	18	12	0	10	170	36
Entenmann's Chocolate Fudge Layer Cake	71g	270	11	4	0	25	230	40
Entenmann's Crumb Topped Cheese Coffee Cake	54g	200	10	4	0	25	160	25
Entenmann's Crumb Topped Coffee Cake	54g	250	11	3.5	0	15	180	33
Entenmann's Crumb Topped Donuts	60g	250	12	6	0	10	210	36
Entenmann's Crumb Topped Raspberry Danish	53g	220	11	4.5	0	15	170	29
Entenmann's Frosted Chocolate Donuts	31g	160	11	7	0	5	90	15
Entenmann's Frosted Softees Assorted Donuts	43g	190	11	5	0	0	210	21
Entenmann's Iced Cheese Danish	57g	230	12	4.5	0	20	200	29
Entenmann's Iced Cinnamon Swirl Buns	85g	320	14	5	0	35	230	45
Entenmann's Little Bites Blueberry Muffins	47g	180	8	1.5	0	25	190	25
Entenmann's Little Bites Chocolate Chip Muffins	47g	190	9	2.5	0	20	135	26
Entenmann's Louisiana Crunch Cake	82g	330	14	4	0	45	300	49
Entenmann's Softees Assorted Donuts	43g	190	11	5	0	0	210	21
Entenmann's Softees Powdered Sugar Donuts	57g	250	12	6	0	25	290	32
Entenmann's Softees Uncoated Donuts	43g	190	11	5	0	0	210	21
Entenmann's Glazed Buttermilk Donuts	64g	270	13	7	0	15	230	37
Entenmann's Glazed Pop'Em Donuts	52g	220	10	5	0	0	170	30
Food For Life Ezekiel 4:9 Sesame Bread	34g	80	0.5	0	0	0	80	14
Food For Life Ezekiel 4:9 Sprouted Grain Bread	34g	80	0.5	0	0	0	75	15
Freihofer D'Italiano White Bread	32g	80	1	0	0	0	240	16

Baked Goods & Doughs

	Serving	Calories	Total fat (gm)	Saturated fat (gm)	Trans fats (gm)	Cholesterol (mg)	Sodium (mg)	Carbs (gm)
Freihofer Original Hamburger Buns	43g	120	1.5	0	0	0	230	23
Freihofer Potato Bread	36g	100	1.5	0	0	0	170	19
Freihofer Wheat Bread	47g	130	2	0	0	0	230	24
Freihofer White Bread	47g	130	1.5	0	0	0	260	24
Freihofer White Hot Dog Buns	43g	120	1.5	0	0	0	240	23
Healthy Choice 7 Grain Bread	38g	80	1	0	0	0	170	18
Healthy Life 100% Whole Wheat Bread	41g	70	0.5	0	0	0	210	16
Heiner's White Bread	26g	70	0.5	0	0	0	210	17
Hillbilly Whole Grain Bread	26g	60	0.5	0	0	0	105	12
Home Pride Wheat Bread	28g	70	1	0	0	0	160	13
Home Pride White Bread	28g	70	1	0	0	0	140	14
Hostess Banana Walnut Muffins	57g	250	16	2.5	0	30	140	25
Hostess Donettes Frosted Chocolate Donuts	61g	270	17	11	0	15	210	29
Hostess Donettes Powdered Sugar Donuts	59g	230	11	5	0	20	230	31
International Fabulous Flats White Naan	63g	160	3.5	1	0	5	480	28
Iron Kids White Bread	26g	60	0.5	0	0	0	120	13
Joseph's White Pita Pockets	41g	80	1	0	0	0	230	16
King's Hawaiian Dinner Rolls	28g	100	2.5	1.5	0	15	80	16
King's Hawaiian Sweet Bread	56g	200	5	3	0	30	160	32
La Tortillas Factory Smart & Delicious Whole Wheat Tortillas	36g	50	2	0	0	0	210	10
Lenders Plain Bagels	81g	210	1.5	0.5	0	0	440	43
Little Debbie Assorted Muffins	54g	210	9	2	0	20	170	28
Little Debbie Blueberry Muffins	54g	190	8	1.5	0	10	170	27
Little Debbie Pecan Spinwheels	28g	100	4	1	0	5	75	16
Little Debbie Powder Sugar Donuts	53g	210	10	5	0	15	220	29
Little Debbie Glazed Honey Buns	50g	220	12	6	0	5	170	26
Little Debbie Glazed Stick Donuts	47g	230	14	7	0	10	160	25
Maier's Italian Bread	1 slice	80	1	0	0	0	0	16
Maier's Italian Steak Rolls	1 roll	170	1	0	0	0	320	31
Martin's Potato Bread	32g	80	1.0	0	0	0	120	15
Martin's Potato Dinner Rolls	35g	90	1.0	0	0	0	130	17
Martin's White Hamburger Rolls	64g	170	3.0	1.0	0	0	280	32
Martin's White Hoagie Rolls	94g	220	3	1	0	0	460	44
Martin's Whole Wheat Potato Bread	35g	70	1.0	0	0	0	125	14
Merita Country 100% Whole Wheat Bread	1 slice	90	1	0	0	0	180	17
Mission Carb Balance Flour Tortillas	42g	110	2.5	0.5	0	0	330	18
Mission Corn Tortillas	49g	130	2	0	0	0	340	25
Mission Flour Tortillas	49g	140	4	1	0	0	460	23

Baked Goods & Doughs

	Serving	Calories	Total fat (gm)	Saturated fat (gm)	Trans fats (gm)	Cholesterol (mg)	Sodium (mg)	Carbs (gm)
Mission Wheat Tortillas	28g	80	2	0	0	0	240	12
Mother's Wheat Bread	28g	80	1	0	0	0	150	14
Mrs. Baird's 100% Whole Wheat Bread	26g	60	1	0	0	0	110	12
Mrs. Baird's 7 Grain Honey Bread	57g	150	2.5	0	0	0	210	26
Mrs. Baird's White Bread	26g	70	1	0	0	0	115	13
Nature's Own 100% Whole Wheat Bread	1 slice	50	1	0	0	0	115	10
Nature's Own 12 Grain Bread	1 slice	90	1	0	0	0	220	20
Nature's Own Butter Bread	1 slice	60	0.5	0	0	0	140	12
Nature's Own Honey 7 Grain Bread	1 slice	60	1	0	0	0	120	13
Nature's Own Honey Wheat Bread	1 slice	60	0.5	0	0	0	125	12
Nature's Own White Wheat Bread	1 slice	55	0.5	0	0	0	115	12
Nature's Pride 100% Whole Wheat Bread	43g	110	1	0	0	0	210	20
Nestle Tollhouse Chocolate Chip Cookie Dough	28g	130	6	2.5	0	5	90	17
Nestle Tollhouse Chocolate Chip Walnut Cookie Dough	39g	180	9	4	0	20	160	23
Nestle Tollhouse Oatmeal Raisin Cookie Dough	39g	160	6	3	0	15	140	24
Nestle Tollhouse Ultimate Chocolate Chip Cookie Dough	38g	180	9	4.5	0	10	150	23
Nestle Tollhouse Ultimate Chocolate Macadamia Nut Cookie Dough	38g	170	9	4.5	0	5	170	22
Nickles Italian Bread	32g	90	1	0	0	0	220	17
Nickles Toastmaster King White Bread	25g	70	0.5	0	0	0	150	14
Nissen Canadian White Bread	39g	100	1.5	0	0	0	190	19
Old El Paso Flour Tortillas	41g	130	4	1	1	0	300	20
Orowheat 100% Whole Wheat Bread	38g	90	1	0	0	0	190	18
Orowheat 100% Whole Wheat Hamburger Buns	74g	180	3	0.5	0	0	370	32
Orowheat 100% Whole Wheat Hot Dog Buns	1 bun	160	2.5	0.5	0	0	320	28
Orowheat 12 Grain Bread	38g	100	1.5	0	0	0	170	18
Orowheat 7 Grain Bread	38g	100	1	0	0	0	180	20
Orowheat Jewish Rye Bread	28g	80	1	0	0	0	170	15
Orowheat Schwazwalder Dark Rye Bread	28g	80	1	0	0	0	210	14
Orowheat Sourdough English Muffins	59g	140	1	0	0	0	240	27
Orowheat Whole Wheat Muffins	59g	130	1.5	0	0	0	240	25
Orowheat Whole Grain & Flax Bread	1 slice	100	1.5	0	0	0	160	17
Orowheat Whole Grain English Muffins	59g	110	1	0	0	0	280	27
Orowheat Whole Grain Oat Bread	1 slice	90	1	0	0	0	180	17
Orowheat Golden Hamburger Buns	74g	200	4.5	1	0	35	360	33

Baked Goods & Doughs	Serving	Calories	Total fat (gm)	Saturated fat (gm)	Trans fats (gm)	Cholesterol (mg)	Sodium (mg)	Carbs (gm)
Pepperidge Farm 100% Stone Ground Whole Wheat Bread	25g	70	1.0	0	0	0	90	12
Pepperidge Farm 100% Whole Wheat Hamburger Rolls	43g	120	2	0	0	0	190	18
Pepperidge Farm Cinnamon Swirl Bread	28g	80	1.5	0	0	0	110	15
Pepperidge Farm Dark Pumpernickel Bread	32g	80	1.0	0	0	0	190	15
Pepperidge Farm Deli Swirl Rye & Pumpernickel Bread	32g	80	1	0	0	0	180	14
Pepperidge Farm Farmhouse 100% Whole Wheat Bread	43g	110	2	0.5	0	0	150	19
Pepperidge Farm Farmhouse 12 Grain Bread	43g	120	2	0	0	0	180	21
Pepperidge Farm Farmhouse Hearty White Bread	43g	120	1.5	0.5	0	0	250	22
Pepperidge Farm Farmhouse Soft Oatmeal Bread	43g	120	1.5	0.5	0	0	200	21
Pepperidge Farm Farmhouse Sourdough Bread	43g	120	1.5	0.5	0	0	220	22
Pepperidge Farm Farmhouse Whole Grain White Bread	43g	110	2	0.5	0	0	180	21
Pepperidge Farm Jewish Rye Bread	32g	80	1	0	0	0	170	15
Pepperidge Farm Light Style 7 Grain Bread	57g	130	1	0	0	0	270	26
Pepperidge Farm Light Style Oatmeal Bread	57g	140	1	0	0	0	260	27
Pepperidge Farm Light Style Wheat Bread	57g	130	1.5	0	0	0	280	26
Pepperidge Farm Mini Plain Bagels	40g	110	0.5	0	0	0	200	22
Pepperidge Farm Natural Whole Grains 100% Whole Wheat Bread	43g	100	2.0	0	0	0	180	20
Pepperidge Farm Natural Whole Grains 15 Grain Bread	43g	120	2	0.5	0	0	180	20
Pepperidge Farm Natural Whole Grains 9 Grain Bread	43g	100	2	0	0	0	180	20
Pepperidge Farm Natural Whole Grains Honey Whole Wheat Bread	43g	110	2	0.5	0	0	170	20
Pepperidge Farm Natural Whole Grains German Wheat Bread	43g	100	1.5	0	0	0	210	20
Pepperidge Farm Plain Bagels	99g	260	1	0	0	0	500	54
Pepperidge Farm Raisin Cinnamon Swirl Bread	28g	80	1.5	0	0	0	100	15
Pepperidge Farm Seedless Rye Bread	32g	80	1	0	0	0	170	14
Pepperidge Farm Very Thin Light White Bread	45g	120	1	0	0	0	250	24
Pepperidge Farm Very Thin Wheat Bread	45g	110	2	0.5	0	0	230	20
Pepperidge Farm White Bread	25g	70	1	0	0	0	100	13
Pepperidge Farm White Hamburger Buns	37g	140	1	0	0	0	530	28
Pepperidge Farm White Hoagie Rolls	69g	200	5	1.5	0	0	320	33

Baked Goods & Doughs

	Serving	Calories	Total fat (gm)	Saturated fat (gm)	Trans fats (gm)	Cholesterol (mg)	Sodium (mg)	Carbs (gm)
Pepperidge Farm White Hot Dog Buns	50g	140	2.5	1	0	0	270	24
Pepperidge Farm White Sandwich Buns	46g	130	3.0	0.5	0	0	220	22
Pepperidge Farm Whole Grain 100% Whole Wheat Bread	43g	100	1.5	0	0	0	170	21
Pepperidge Farm Whole Grain Oatmeal Bread	43g	110	2	0.5	0	0	170	20
Pillsbury Big Deluxe Classic Chocolate Chip Cookie Dough	38g	170	9	3	2	10	125	22
Pillsbury Big Deluxe Classic Oatmeal Raisin Cookie Dough	38g	160	6	1.5	1.5	10	100	23
Pillsbury Biscuits	64g	150	2	0	0	0	570	29
Pillsbury Breadsticks	52g	140	2.5	1	0	0	360	25
Pillsbury Butter Crescent Rolls	48g	170	9	2.5	2.5	0	370	20
Pillsbury Butter Dinner Rolls	48g	170	9	2.5	2.5	0	370	20
Pillsbury Butterflake Dinner Rolls	28g	110	6	2	1.5	0	220	11
Pillsbury Buttermilk Biscuits	64g	150	2	0	0	0	570	29
Pillsbury Chocolate Chip Cookie Dough	29g	130	7	2.5	1.5	5	95	18
Pillsbury Cinnamon Rolls	49g	170	6	1.5	2.5	0	370	26
Pillsbury Cinnamon Twists	46g	180	9	2.5	2.5	0	310	22
Pillsbury Create N' Bake Chocolate Chip Cookie Dough	29g	130	7	2.5	1.5	5	95	18
Pillsbury Create N' Bake Peanut Butter Cookie Dough	29g	130	6	1.5	1	5	135	16
Pillsbury Create N' Bake Sugar Cookie Dough	29g	130	6	1.5	1.5	10	95	18
Pillsbury Crescent Rolls	28g	90	4.5	1.5	0	0	220	12
Pillsbury Dinner Rolls	28g	110	6	2	1.5	0	220	11
Pillsbury French Bread Dough	52g	120	1.5	0.5	0	0	300	24
Pillsbury Orange Sweet Rolls	49g	170	6	1.5	1.5	0	340	26
Pillsbury Pie Crust	27g	110	7	2.5	0	5	140	12
Pillsbury Pizza Crust	62g	180	5	1	0	0	360	29
Pillsbury Place N' Bake Crescent Rolls	28g	110	6	2	1.5	0	220	11
Pillsbury Ready To Bake Chocolate Chip Cookie Dough	38g	170	9	3	2	10	125	22
Pillsbury Ready To Bake Chunky Chocolate Chip Cookie Dough	38g	180	9	3	2	10	125	22
Pillsbury Ready To Bake Oatmeal Chocolate Chip Cookie Dough	38g	170	8	2.5	1.5	10	95	23
Pillsbury Ready To Bake Sugar Cookie Dough	38g	170	9	2.5	2.5	10	100	22
Pillsbury Recipe Creations Crescent Rolls	38g	120	6	2.5	0	0	300	16
Pillsbury Garlic Butter Dinner Rolls	28g	110	6	2	1.5	0	260	11
Pillsbury Golden Layers Butter Tastin' Biscuits	34g	110	4	1	1	0	360	14

Baked Goods & Doughs

	Serving	Calories	Total fat (gm)	Saturated fat (gm)	Trans fats (gm)	Cholesterol (mg)	Sodium (mg)	Carbs (gm)
Pillsbury Golden Layers Buttermilk Biscuits	34g	110	4	1	1	0	360	14
Pillsbury Golden Layers Honey Butter Biscuits	34g	110	4	1	1	0	290	15
Pillsbury Grands Biscuits	58g	160	6	2	0	0	590	26
Pillsbury Grands Butter Biscuits	58g	180	8	2.5	3	0	580	25
Pillsbury Grands Buttermilk Biscuits	58g	160	6	3.5	0	0	590	25
Pillsbury Grands Cinnamon Rolls	99g	370	19	5	5	0	650	48
Pillsbury Grands Original Biscuits	58g	170	7	1.5	3	0	580	24
Sara Lee 100% Whole Wheat Bread	57g	150	2	0.5	0	0	270	26
Sara Lee Blueberry Bagels	104g	290	1.5	0	0	0	430	61
Sara Lee Butter Dinner Rolls	40g	110	1.5	0.5	0	0	190	21
Sara Lee Cinnamon Raisin Bagels	104g	280	1.5	0	0	0	520	60
Sara Lee Delightful 100% Multigrain Bread	45g	90	1.5	0	0	0	210	18
Sara Lee Delightful 100% Whole Wheat Bread	45g	90	1	0	0	0	210	18
Sara Lee Delightful 45 Calorie Wheat Bread	45g	90	1	0	0	0	230	18
Sara Lee Heart Healthy 100% Whole Wheat Hamburger Buns	74g	210	3	1	0	0	360	35
Sara Lee Hearty & Delicious 100% Multigrain Bread	43g	120	1.5	0.5	0	0	210	20
Sara Lee Hearty & Delicious 100% Whole Wheat Bread	43g	120	1.5	0.5	0	0	210	21
Sara Lee Hearty & Delicious 100% Whole Wheat Bread with Honey	43g	110	1.5	0.5	0	0	210	21
Sara Lee Honey Wheat Bread	28g	80	1	0	0	0	140	14
Sara Lee Plain Bagels	37g	100	0.5	0	0	0	190	21
Sara Lee Soft & Smooth 100% Whole Wheat Bread	28g	70	1	0	0	0	135	12
Sara Lee Soft & Smooth Classic White Bread	57g	160	2	0	0	0	300	30
Sara Lee Soft & Smooth Honey Wheat Bread	57g	150	2.5	0.5	0	0	260	26
Sara Lee Soft & Smooth Wheat Hamburger Buns	43g	120	2	0.5	0	0	220	22
Sara Lee Soft & Smooth Wheat Hot Dog Buns	43g	120	2	0.5	0	0	220	22
Sara Lee Soft & Smooth Whole Grain Honey Wheat Bread	57g	160	2	1	0	5	260	29
Sara Lee Soft & Smooth Whole Grain White Bread	57g	150	2	1	0	5	250	28
Sara Lee Soft & Smooth Whole Grain White Hamburger Buns	43g	120	1.5	0.5	0	0	220	22
Sara Lee White Hamburger Buns	74g	200	2	0	0	0	380	39
Sara Lee White Hoagie Rolls	76g	200	2	0.5	0	0	400	39
Sara Lee White Hot Dog Buns	43g	120	1.5	0.5	0	0	220	22

Baked Goods & Doughs

	Serving	Calories	Total fat (gm)	Saturated fat (gm)	Trans fats (gm)	Cholesterol (mg)	Sodium (mg)	Carbs (gm)
Sara Lee Whole Grain White Hot Dog Buns	43g	120	1.5	0.5	0	0	220	22
Schwebels White Bread	1 slice	80	1	0	0	0	140	16
Soft N' Good White Bread	1 slice	80	1	0	0	0	140	16
Stroehmann Dutch Country 100% Whole Wheat Bread	1 slice	100	1.5	0	0	0	200	18
Stroehmann Dutch Country Potato Bread	1 slice	100	1.5	0	0	0	170	18
Stroehmann Wheat Bread	1 slice	90	1	0	0	0	180	18
Stroehmann White Bread	1 slice	65	0.75	0	0	0	125	12
Stroehmann White Hamburger Buns	1 bun	110	1.5	0	0	0	210	21
Sunbeam White Bread	1 slice	55	0.75	0	0	0	140	11
Sun-Maid Cinnamon Swirl Bread	32g	100	1.5	0.5	0	5	115	18
Thomas' 100% Whole Wheat Bagels	43g	110	1	0	0	0	180	22
Thomas' Blueberry Bagels	104g	300	2.5	1	0	0	470	60
Thomas' Cinnamon Raisin Bagels	43g	120	1.0	0	0	0	210	24
Thomas' Cinnamon Raisin English Muffins	61g	140	1	0	0	0	170	29
Thomas' Cinnamon Raisin Swirl Bagels	95g	250	1.5	0.5	0	0	410	49
Thomas' Cinnamon Swirl Bagels	104g	300	3	1.5	0	0	500	57
Thomas' Cornbread Muffins	33g	110	3.5	0.5	0	5	190	17
Thomas' Everything Bagels	104g	300	4	1	0	0	510	54
Thomas' Hearty Grains 100% Whole Wheat English Muffins	57g	120	1.0	0	0	0	220	23
Thomas' Hearty Grains Honey Oatmeal Bagels	95g	270	2.5	0.5	0	0	420	53
Thomas' Hearty Grains Honey Oatmeal English Muffins	57g	130	1.0	0	0	0	180	25
Thomas' Hearty Grains Honey Wheat English Muffins	57g	120	0.5	0	0	0	220	27
Thomas' Hearty Grains Multigrain English Muffins	57g	150	2.5	0	0	0	160	27
Thomas' Multigrain Fork Split English Muffins	57g	100	1.0	0	0	0	190	24
Thomas' Onion Bagels	95g	260	2	0.5	0	0	470	51
Thomas' Original English Muffins	57g	130	1	0	0	0	220	26
Thomas' Plain Bagels	104g	290	2	0.5	0	0	540	56
Thomas' Plain Fork Split English Muffins	57g	120	1.0	0	0	0	200	25
Thomas' Plain Whole Grain Bagels	95g	260	2	0.5	0	0	470	51
Thomas' Sahara 100% Whole Wheat Pita Pockets	57g	140	1.5	0	0	0	310	27
Thomas' Whole Wheat Bagels	104g	270	2	1	0	0	440	55
Village Hearth Cottage Bread	34g	80	1	0	0	0	180	15
Weight Watchers Blueberry Muffins	66g	190	2.5	0.5	0	15	370	42
Wonder 100% Whole Wheat Bread	32g	80	1.0	0	0	0	170	14

Baked Goods & Doughs

Baked Goods & Doughs	Serving	Calories	Total fat (gm)	Saturated fat (gm)	Trans fats (gm)	Cholesterol (mg)	Sodium (mg)	Carbs (gm)
Wonder 100% Whole Grain White Bread	31g	80	1.0	0	0	0	150	15
Wonder Hot Dog Buns	43g	110	1.5	0	0	0	210	21
Wonder Kids White Bread	26g	60	0.5	0	0	0	115	12
Wonder Wheat Light Bread	45g	80	0.5	0	0	0	240	18
Wonder White Bread	1 slice	110	1.5	0	0	0	230	20
Wonder White Hamburger Buns	43g	110	1.5	0	0	0	210	21
Wonder Whole Grain Wheat Bread	57g	130	1.5	0	0	0	320	26

Grocery Food Factoid:

The safe amount of trans fats to eat is 0 grams. These four popcorn products have over 5 grams per serving!

Pop Secret Butter Microwave Popcorn

Pop Secret Movie Theater Butter Microwave Popcorn

Pop Secret Extra Butter Microwave Popcorn

Pop Secret Salted Homestyle Butter Microwave Popcorn

SHOPPING LIST/NOTES:

_____

_____

_____

_____

_____

_____

_____

_____

_____

_____

_____

_____

_____

_____

_____

_____

_____

_____

_____

_____

_____

_____

Baking Items

	Serving	Calories	Total fat (gm)	Saturated fat (gm)	Trans fats (gm)	Cholesterol (mg)	Sodium (mg)	Carbs (gm)
123 Vegetable Oil	14g	126	14	1.2	0	0	0	0
100% Whole Wheat Flour	1 cup	407	2	0	0	0	6	87
Baker's Semisweet Chocolate Squares	14g	70	4.5	2.5	0	0	0	8
Baker's Unsweetened Chocolate Squares	14g	70	7	4.5	0	0	0	4
Bertolli Olive Oil	15ml	120	14	2	0	0	0	0
Betty Crocker Bacos Bacon Bits	7g	30	1.5	0	0	0	115	2
Betty Crocker Brownie Mix	30g	120	2.5	1	0	0	90	25
Betty Crocker Cookie Mix	27g	120	3	1.5	0	0	105	21
Betty Crocker Muffin Mix	30g	120	2.5	0.5	1	0	230	23
Betty Crocker Pizza Crust Mix	46g	160	2	0	0	0	340	33
Betty Crocker Ready To Spread Frosting	33g	130	5	1.5	2	0	95	21
Betty Crocker Supermoist Cake Mix	43g	170	2.5	0.5	0.5	0	280	35
Betty Crocker Ultimate Fudge Brownie Mix	30g	120	2	1	0	0	95	24
Betty Crocker Walnut Fudge Brownie Mix	28g	120	3	0.5	0	0	90	22
Betty Crocker Warm Delights Hot Fudge Brownie Mix	88g	370	12	4.5	2	0	270	61
Betty Crocker White Angel Food Cake Mix	38g	140	0	0	0	0	320	32
Betty Crocker Whipped Ready To Spread Frosting	24g	100	5	1.5	1.5	0	45	15
Bisquick Heart Smart All Purpose Baking Mix	40g	140	2.5	0	0	0	340	27
Bisquick Original All Purpose Baking Mix	40g	160	5	1.5	1.5	0	490	26
Boboli Pizza Crust	47g	120	2.5	1	0	0	230	22
Borden Eagle Fat Free Sweetened Condensed Milk	39g	110	0	0	0	5	40	24
Borden Eagle Sweetened Condensed Milk	39g	130	3	2	0	10	40	23
Brown Sugar	10g	38	0	0	0	0	0	10
C&H Dark Brown Pure Cane Sugar	4g	15	0	0	0	0	0	4
C&H White Powdered Sugar	30g	120	0	0	0	0	0	30
C&H Golden Brown Pure Cane Sugar	4g	15	0	0	0	0	0	4
C&H Granulated White Sugar	4g	15	0	0	0	0	0	4
Canola Oil	36g	130	15	1	0	0	0	0
Carapelli Extra Virgin Olive Oil	36g	130	14	2	0	0	310	0
Chef Boyardee Cheese Pizza Kit	113g	250	4	1.5	0	5	730	45
Colavita Extra Virgin Olive Oil	15ml	120	14	2	0	0	0	0
Comstock Cherry Pie & Pastry Filling	89g	90	0	0	0	0	25	23
Crisco Canola Oil	14g	120	14	1	0	0	0	0
Crisco Extra Virgin Olive Oil	14g	120	14	2	0	0	0	0
Crisco Vegetable Oil	14g	120	14	2	0	0	0	0
Crisco Vegetable Shortening	12g	110	12	3	0	0	0	0
Diamond Unsalted Chopped Pecans	30g	210	22	2	0	0	0	4

Baking Items

Baking Items	Serving	Calories	Total fat (gm)	Saturated fat (gm)	Trans fats (gm)	Cholesterol (mg)	Sodium (mg)	Carbs (gm)
Diamond Unsalted Chopped Walnuts	30g	200	20	2	0	0	0	4
Domino Dark Brown Sugar	4g	15	0	0	0	0	0	4
Domino Light Brown Sugar	4g	15	0	0	0	0	0	4
Domino Powdered Sugar	30g	120	0	0	0	0	0	30
Domino Granulated White Sugar	4g	15	0	0	0	0	0	4
Duncan Hines Brownie Mix	30g	120	2.5	0.5	0	0	115	24
Duncan Hines Chocolate Lover's Double Fudge Brownie Mix	31g	130	2.5	0.5	0.5	0	110	26
Duncan Hines Chocolate Lover's Walnut Brownie Mix	31g	130	3.5	0.5	0	0	110	24
Duncan Hines Creamy Homestyle Frosting	35g	140	6	1.5	1.5	0	95	22
Duncan Hines Moist Deluxe Cake Mix	52g	230	5	2	0.5	0	230	43
Durkee Marshmallow Fluff	12g	40	0	0	0	0	5	10
Filippo Berio Olive Oil	15ml	120	14	2	0	0	0	0
Ghirardelli Double Chocolate Brownie Mix	35g	140	3.5	1.5	0	0	120	27
Ghirardelli Double Chocolate Chips	15g	80	6	3.5	0	0	0	8
Ghirardelli Unsweetened Milk Chocolate Chips	15g	70	3.5	2.5	0	0	10	10
Jello Flavored Pudding/Pie Filling Mix	25g	90	0	0	0	0	360	23
Jello No-Bake Cheesecake	53g	220	5	3	0	0	370	42
Jello Sugar Free Flavored Pudding/Pie Filling Mix	8g	25	0	0	0	0	300	6
Keebler Pie Crust	21g	100	3.5	1	1.5	0	100	15
Kraft Marshmallow Cream	13g	40	0	0	0	0	10	11
Libby's Pure Pumpkin Pie Filling	87g	90	0.5	0	0	0	120	20
Lou Ana Peanut Oil	14g	120	14	2.5	0	0	0	0
Mazola Canola Oil	14g	120	14	1	0	0	0	0
Mazola Corn Oil	14g	120	14	2	0	0	0	0
Mazola Vegetable Plus Canola Oil	14g	120	14	2	0	0	0	0
Minute Tapioca Pudding/Pie Filling Mix	6g	20	0	0	0	0	0	5
Nestle Carnation Sweetened Condensed Milk	40g	130	3	2	0	10	45	22
Nestle La Lechera Plain Sweetened Condensed Milk	30ml	130	3	2	0	10	45	22
Olive Oil	14g	120	14	2	0	0	0	0
Oven-Fry Seasoned Coating Mix	15g	60	1	0	0	0	330	11
Pam Canola Oil Non-Stick Cooking Spray	0g	0	0	0	0	0	0	0
Pam Vegetable Oil Non-Stick Cooking Spray	15ml	0	0	0	0	0	0	0
Pillsbury Banana Bread Baking Mix	28g	110	1	0	0	0	160	22
Pillsbury Chocolate Fudge Brownie Mix	28g	110	2.5	0	0	0	85	23

Baking Items

	Serving	Calories	Total fat (gm)	Saturated fat (gm)	Trans fats (gm)	Cholesterol (mg)	Sodium (mg)	Carbs (gm)
Pillsbury Creamy Supreme Ready To Spread Frosting	35g	140	6	1.5	2	0	90	21
Pillsbury Funfetti Premium Cake Mix	45g	180	3.5	1.5	0	0	300	36
Pillsbury Milk Chocolate Brownie Mix	28g	110	2	0	0	0	70	23
Pillsbury Moist Supreme Cake Mix	43g	160	2.5	1	0	0	330	35
Pompeian Extra Virgin Olive Oil	14g	120	14	2	0	0	0	0
Powdered Sugar	120g	467	0.1	0	0	0	1	119
Progresso Breadcrumbs	28g	110	1.5	0.5	0	0	200	20
Ragu Pizza Sauce	63g	40	2	0	0	0	380	6
Shake & Bake Seasoned Coating Mix	11g	40	0	0	0	0	240	8
Shortening	12g	110	12	3	0	0	0	0
Smart Balance Canola Soy & Olive Oil	120	120	14	1.5	0	0	0	0
Star Extra Virgin Olive Oil	14g	120	14	2	0	0	0	0
Sugar	1 cup	774	0	0	0	0	0	200
Sugar in The Raw Blond Sugar	4g	15	0	0	0	0	0	4
Vegetable Oil	15ml	120	14	1	0	0	0	0
Wesson Canola Oil	15ml	120	14	1	0	0	0	0
Wesson Corn Oil	15ml	120	14	2	0	0	0	0
Wesson Vegetable Oil	15ml	120	14	2	0	0	0	0
White Flour Bleached	1 cup	11	1.2	0	0	0	3	96
White Flour Unbleached	1 cup	16	2	0	0	0	3	104
White Whole Wheat Flour	1 cup	456	1	0	0	0	4	96
Wilderness Country Cherry Pie & Pastry Filling	89g	90	0	0	0	0	25	23

Grocery Food Factoid:

The world can be divided into two groups: those who like soda and those who don't. In this guide soda with sugar is colored red and diet sodas are colored yellow. This is different from the yellow color they get in the Fast Food Guide (www.fastfoodbook.com). This is because a different scoring system was used. Either way, don't drink too much soda. Pick something green instead.

SHOPPING LIST/NOTES:

_____
_____
_____
_____
_____
_____

Beverages

Beverages	Serving	Calories	Total fat (gm)	Saturated fat (gm)	Trans fats (gm)	Cholesterol (mg)	Sodium (mg)	Carbs (gm)
7-UP Lemon Lime Soda	244ml	100	0	0	0	0	25	26
A&W Cream Soda	244ml	130	0	0	0	0	45	32
A&W Diet Caffeine Free Root Beer	355ml	0	0	0	0	0	100	0
A&W Diet Root Beer	240ml	0	0	0	0	0	70	0
A&W Root Beer	254ml	120	0	0	0	0	45	32
AMP Energy Drink	240ml	110	0	0	0	0	65	29
AMP Overdrive Cherry Energy Drink	240ml	110	0	0	0	0	70	29
Apple & Eve Apple Juice from Concentrate	248ml	110	0	0	0	0	5	26
Barq's Root Beer	355ml	160	0	0	0	0	70	45
Big Red Cream Soda	239ml	100	0	0	0	0	20	25
Big Red Soda	360ml	150	0	0	0	0	30	38
Bolthouse Farms C Boost Tropical Fruit Juice Smoothie	230ml	152	0	0	0	0	15	36
Bolthouse Farms Carrot Juice	244ml	70	0	0	0	0	150	14
Bolthouse Farms Green Goodness Juice	240ml	140	0	0	0	0	25	33
Caffeine Free Coke	240ml	100	0	0	0	0	35	27
Caffeine Free Diet Coke	355ml	0	0	0	0	0	40	0
Caffeine Free Diet Pepsi	355ml	0	0	0	0	0	35	0
Caffeine Free Pepsi	240ml	100	0	0	0	0	20	28
Campbell's Tomato Juice	240ml	50	0	0	0	0	680	10
Canada Dry Ginger Ale	244ml	90	0	0	0	0	35	25
Capri Sun Assorted Juices	200ml	70	0	0	0	0	15	19
Cherry 7-Up Cherry Lemon Lime Soda	244ml	100	0	0	0	0	25	26
Cherry Coke	240ml	100	0	0	0	0	25	28
Cherry Coke Zero	240ml	0	0	0	0	0	30	0
Citrus Mountain Dew	240ml	110	0	0	0	0	0	31
Code Red Mountain Dew	244ml	110	0	0	0	0	70	31
Coke Classic	240ml	100	0	0	0	0	35	27
Coke Zero	355ml	0	0	0	0	0	40	0
Daily's Little Hugs Assorted Drinks	244ml	35	0	0	0	0	90	8
Diet 7-Up Lemon Lime Soda	240ml	0	0	0	0	0	30	0
Diet Cherry Coke	355ml	0	0	0	0	0	40	0
Diet Coke	240ml	0	0	0	0	0	30	0
Diet Coke with Lime	355ml	0	0	0	0	0	40	0
Diet Coke with Splenda	355ml	0	0	0	0	0	40	0
Diet Dr Pepper	240ml	0	0	0	0	0	35	0
Diet Mountain Dew	355ml	0	0	0	0	0	50	0
Diet Mountain Dew Code Red	355ml	0	0	0	0	0	40	0
Diet Pepsi	240ml	0	0	0	0	0	25	0
Diet Pepsi Max	355ml	0	0	0	0	0	35	0

Beverages

Beverages	Serving	Calories	Total fat (gm)	Saturated fat (gm)	Trans fats (gm)	Cholesterol (mg)	Sodium (mg)	Carbs (gm)
Diet Pepsi Vanilla	355ml	0	0	0	0	0	35	0
Diet Rite	240ml	0	0	0	0	0	0	0
Diet Rite Pure Zero	355ml	0	0	0	0	0	0	0
Diet Schweppes Ginger Ale	240ml	0	0	0	0	0	80	0
Diet Sunkist Orange Soda	240ml	0	0	0	0	0	80	0
Diet V-8 Splash Fruit Juice	240ml	10	0	0	0	0	25	3
Diet Wild Cherry Pepsi	355ml	0	0	0	0	0	35	0
Dole Orange Peach Mango Juice	250g	120	0	0	0	0	25	29
Dole Organic Strawberry Banana Juice	243g	120	0	0	0	0	10	30
Dole Paradise Blend Juice	250ml	120	0	0	0	0	40	29
Dole Pina Colada Juice	248ml	120	0	0	0	0	10	29
Dole Pineapple Juice	250g	130	0	0	0	0	10	30
Dole Pineapple Orange Banana Juice	250ml	120	0	0	0	0	10	30
Dole Pineapple Orange Juice	250g	120	0	0	0	0	10	31
Dole Strawberry Kiwi Juice	240ml	120	0	0	0	0	25	31
Dr. Pepper	240ml	100	0	0	0	0	35	27
Fanta Caffeine Free Orange Soda	361ml	160	0	0	0	0	55	44
Fanta Orange Soda	240ml	110	0	0	0	0	35	30
Florida's Natural Orange Juice	240ml	110	0	0	0	0	0	26
Florida's Natural Orange Juice No Pulp	249ml	110	0	0	0	0	0	26
Florida's Natural Orange Juice with Calcium & Vitamin D	240ml	110	0	0	0	0	0	26
Florida's Natural Orange Juice with Pulp	249ml	110	0	0	0	0	0	26
Florida's Natural Orange Juice with Pulp, Calcium, & Vitamin C	249ml	110	0	0	0	0	0	26
Florida's Natural Ruby Red Grapefruit Juice	247g	90	0	0	0	0	0	22
Fresca Diet Black Cherry Citrus Soda	355ml	0	0	0	0	0	35	0
Fresca Diet Peach Citrus Soda	355ml	0	0	0	0	0	35	0
Fresca Diet Grapefruit Soda	355ml	0	0	0	0	0	35	0
Full Throttle Energy Drink	473ml	220	0	0	0	0	160	57
Fuze Refresh Fruit Drink	248ml	90	0	0	0	0	15	25
Fuze Slenderize Fruit Drink	240ml	5	0	0	0	0	5	2
G2 Flavored Sports Drink	248ml	25	0	0	0	0	110	7
Gatorade All Stars Flavored Thirst Quencher	355ml	80	0	0	0	0	160	21
Gatorade Drink Mix	16g	60	0	0	0	0	110	16
Gatorade Flavored Sports Drink	240ml	50	0	0	0	0	110	14
Gatorade Flavored Thirst Quencher	240ml	50	0	0	0	0	110	14
Hawaiian Punch Assorted Drinks	240ml	80	0	0	0	0	105	22
Hi-C Assorted Drinks	208ml	100	0	0	0	0	15	27

Beverages

Beverages	Serving	Calories	Total fat (gm)	Saturated fat (gm)	Trans fats (gm)	Cholesterol (mg)	Sodium (mg)	Carbs (gm)
IBC Caffeine Free Root Beer	361ml	160	0	0	0	0	65	44
Java Monster Energy Drink	243ml	100	1.5	1.1	0	0	350	17
Kool-Aid Bursts Flavored Drink	194ml	100	0	0	0	0	30	24
Kool-Aid Jammers Flavored Juice	207ml	90	0	0	0	0	15	24
Martinelli's Gold Medal Sparkling Apple Grape Juice	248ml	120	0	0	0	0	14	31
Minute-Maid Apple Juice	207ml	100	0	0	0	0	15	23
Minute-Maid Apple Juice from Concentrate	295ml	140	0	0	0	0	25	35
Minute-Maid Canned Fruit Punch	355ml	170	0	0	0	0	50	46
Minute-Maid Canned Lemonade	240ml	100	0	0	0	0	35	28
Minute-Maid Canned Light Lemonade	355ml	10	0	0	0	0	120	2
Minute-Maid Canned Pink Lemonade	355ml	150	0	0	0	0	50	42
Minute-Maid Coolers Fruit Punch	206ml	100	0	0	0	0	15	26
Minute-Maid Fruit Punch	206ml	100	0	0	0	0	15	24
Minute-Maid Heart Wise Orange Juice	249ml	110	0	0	0	0	20	27
Minute-Maid Kids Plus Orange Juice	208ml	100	0	0	0	0	15	23
Minute-Maid Light Lemonade	248ml	15	0	0	0	0	15	4
Minute-Maid Mixed Berry Juice	206ml	100	0	0	0	0	15	25
Minute-Maid Multi-Vitamin Orange Juice	249ml	120	0	0	0	0	20	27
Minute-Maid Orange Juice	306ml	140	0	0	0	0	20	33
Minute-Maid Pomegranate Blueberry Juice	240ml	120	0.5	0	0	0	20	31
Minute-Maid Pomegranate Lemonade	248ml	110	0	0	0	0	20	31
Minute-Maid Pomegranate Tea	240ml	100	0	0	0	0	20	28
Minute-Maid Premium Berry Punch	240ml	120	0	0	0	0	15	32
Minute-Maid Premium Cherry Limeade	248ml	120	0	0	0	0	15	34
Minute-Maid Premium For Kids Orange Juice	249ml	110	0	0	0	0	20	27
Minute-Maid Premium Fruit Punch	240ml	120	0	0	0	0	15	31
Minute-Maid Premium High Pulp Orange Juice with Calcium & Vitamin D	249ml	110	0	0	0	0	15	27
Minute-Maid Premium Lemonade	247ml	110	0	0	0	0	15	31
Minute-Maid Premium Light Orange Juice	249ml	50	0	0	0	0	15	13
Minute-Maid Premium Low Pulp Orange Juice	249ml	110	0	0	0	0	15	27
Minute-Maid Premium Low Pulp Orange Juice with Calcium & Vitamin D	249ml	110	0	0	0	0	20	27
Minute-Maid Premium Low-Acid Orange Juice	249ml	110	0	0	0	0	20	27
Minute-Maid Premium Medium Pulp Orange Juice	249ml	110	0	0	0	0	15	27
Minute-Maid Premium Orange Juice with Calcium & Vitamin D	240ml	110	0	0	0	0	20	27

Beverages

Beverages	Serving	Calories	Total fat (gm)	Saturated fat (gm)	Trans fats (gm)	Cholesterol (mg)	Sodium (mg)	Carbs (gm)
Minute-Maid Premium Pink Lemonade	248ml	110	0	0	0	0	15	30
Minute-Maid Premium Pulp Free Orange Juice	249ml	110	0	0	0	0	15	27
Monster Energy Drink	237ml	10	0	0	0	0	180	3
Mott's Apple Juice	240ml	110	0	0	0	0	10	27
Mott's Apple Juice from Concentrate	232ml	120	0	0	0	0	10	29
Mott's Clamato Tomato Juice Cocktail	237ml	60	0	0	0	0	880	11
Mott's For Tots Apple Juice	240ml	60	0	0	0	0	10	15
Mott's Plus Apple Juice	240ml	60	0	0	0	0	35	15
Mountain Dew	361ml	170	0	0	0	0	65	46
Mountain Dew Live Wire	361ml	170	0	0	0	0	65	47
Mug Root Beer	240ml	100	0	0	0	0	40	29
Nestle Juicy Juice Fruit Juice	232ml	120	0	0	0	0	20	29
Nestle Juicy Juice Fruit Juice from Concentrate	248ml	110	0	0	0	0	20	28
Nestle Juicy Juice Harvest Surprise Fruit Juice	253ml	120	0	0	0	0	80	28
Newman's Own Virgin Lemonade	236ml	110	0	0	0	0	40	27
Northland Cranberry Juice	253ml	130	0	0	0	0	35	33
Northland Cranberry Pomegranate Juice	245ml	140	0	0	0	0	25	34
Ocean Spray Cran-Apple Juice	245ml	140	0	0	0	0	80	35
Ocean Spray Cranberry Blueberry Juice	245ml	140	0	0	0	0	35	36
Ocean Spray Cranberry Juice	253ml	140	0	0	0	0	35	35
Ocean Spray Cran-Cherry Juice	240ml	120	0	0	0	0	35	30
Ocean Spray Cran-Grape Juice	245ml	140	0	0	0	0	80	35
Ocean Spray Cran-Raspberry Juice	245ml	120	0	0	0	0	70	30
Ocean Spray Diet Cranberry Juice	236ml	5	0	0	0	0	50	2
Ocean Spray Diet Cranberry Grape Juice	245ml	5	0	0	0	0	50	2
Ocean Spray Light Cranberry Juice Cocktail	238ml	40	0	0	0	0	75	10
Ocean Spray Light Cran-Grape Juice	237ml	40	0	0	0	0	75	10
Ocean Spray Light Cran-Raspberry Juice	237ml	40	0	0	0	0	70	10
Ocean Spray Light Ruby Red Grapefruit Juice	247ml	40	0	0	0	0	65	10
Ocean Spray Ruby Red Grapefruit Juice	247ml	130	0	0	0	0	35	32
Ocean Spray White Cranberry Strawberry Juice	245ml	120	0	0	0	0	50	31
Ocean Spray White Cran-Peach Juice	245ml	120	0	0	0	0	50	31
Ocean Spray White Grapefruit Juice	247ml	90	0	0	0	0	35	21
Odwalla Blueberry B Monster Drink Smoothie	243ml	140	0	0	0	0	10	34
Odwalla Carrot Juice	236ml	70	0	0	0	0	160	15
Odwalla Orange Juice	249ml	110	0	0	0	0	15	25

Beverages

	Serving	Calories	Total fat (gm)	Saturated fat (gm)	Trans fats (gm)	Cholesterol (mg)	Sodium (mg)	Carbs (gm)
Odwalla Strawberry C Monster Drink Smoothie	243ml	160	0	0	0	0	20	38
Odwalla Superfood Juice	248ml	130	0.5	0	0	0	10	30
Old Orchard Apple Juice from Concentrate	244ml	120	0	0	0	0	25	29
Passion Fruit Rockstar Energy Drink	240ml	110	0	0	0	0	30	25
Pepsi	240ml	100	0	0	0	0	20	28
Pepsi One	240ml	1	0	0	0	0	25	0
Pibb Xtra	361ml	140	0	0	0	0	40	39
Pom Wonderful Pomegranate Juice	246ml	150	0	0	0	0	0	40
Powerade Flavored Sports Drink	244ml	60	0	0	0	0	55	17
Powerade Zero Flavored Sports Drink	240ml	0	0	0	0	0	55	0
Propel Flavored Drink Mix	3g	10	0	0	0	0	30	3
RC Cola	236ml	110	0	0	0	0	30	29
Red Bull Energy Drink	249ml	10	0	0	0	0	200	3
Rockstar Energy Drink	240ml	100	0	0	0	0	110	0
RW Knudsen Family Just Cranberry Juice	240ml	70	0	0	0	0	30	18
Schweppes Club Soda	301ml	0	0	0	0	0	80	0
Schweppes Tonic Water	244ml	90	0	0	0	0	35	23
Schweppes Ginger Ale	244ml	80	0	0	0	0	40	23
Seagrams Ginger Ale	240ml	100	0	0	0	0	35	24
Sierra Mist Free Lemon Lime Soda	250ml	0	0	0	0	0	25	0
Sierra Mist Lemon Lime Soda	361ml	140	0	0	0	0	35	39
Simply Apple Juice	240ml	120	0	0	0	0	5	30
Simply Lemonade	248ml	120	0	0	0	0	15	30
Simply Limeade	248ml	120	0	0	0	0	15	31
Simply Orange Juice	249ml	110	0	0	0	0	0	26
Simply Orange Juice Pulp Free	415ml	190	0	0	0	0	0	45
Simply Orange Juice Pulp Free with Calcium	249ml	110	0	0	0	0	0	26
Simply Orange Juice with Calcium	249ml	110	0	0	0	0	0	26
Simply Orange Juice with Pulp	240ml	10	0	0	0	0	0	26
Simply Orange Mango Juice	240ml	120	0	0	0	0	0	28
Simply Orange Pineapple Juice	240ml	110	0	0	0	0	0	27
Simply Grapefruit Juice	247ml	90	0	0	0	0	10	21
Sobe Energy Citrus Drink	244ml	120	0	0	0	0	15	32
Sobe No Fear Energy Drink	240ml	130	0	0	0	0	115	36
Sprite	244ml	100	0	0	0	0	45	26
Sprite Zero	240ml	0	0	0	0	0	25	0
Squirt	254ml	100	0	0	0	0	35	26
Squirt Citrus Burst	361ml	140	0	0	0	0	50	39

Beverages

Beverages	Serving	Calories	Total fat (gm)	Saturated fat (gm)	Trans fats (gm)	Cholesterol (mg)	Sodium (mg)	Carbs (gm)
Sunkist Orange Soda	361ml	190	0	0	0	0	45	52
Sunny Delight	248ml	90	0	0	0	0	170	22
Sunsweet Plum Smart Light Plum Juice Cocktail	240ml	60	0	0	0	0	20	15
Sunsweet Plum Smart Prune Juice	240ml	160	0	0	0	0	55	36
Sunsweet Prune Juice	174ml	120	0	0	0	0	20	30
Tab Cola	355ml	0	0	0	0	0	40	0
Tampico Flavored Punch	248ml	120	0	0	0	0	65	29
Trop 50 Orange Juice	249ml	50	0	0	0	0	10	13
Tropicana Flavored Punch	248ml	130	0	0	0	0	15	32
Tropicana Light Lemonade	244ml	5	0	0	0	0	65	1
Tropicana Pure Pomegranate Blueberry Juice	240ml	130	0	0	0	0	25	33
Tropicana Pure Premium Antioxidant Orange Juice	249g	110	0	0	0	0	0	26
Tropicana Pure Premium Healthy Heart Orange Juice	249ml	120	0.5	0	0	0	0	26
Tropicana Pure Premium Healthy Kids Orange Juice	249ml	110	0	0	0	0	0	26
Tropicana Pure Premium Light 'N Healthy Orange Juice	248ml	50	0	0	0	0	10	13
Tropicana Pure Premium Orange Juice with Calcium & Vitamin D	240ml	110	0	0	0	0	0	26
Tropicana Pure Premium Orange Juice with Calcium, & Vitamins A & C	249g	110	0	0	0	0	0	26
Tropicana Pure Premium Orange Juice with Calcium, Vitamin D & No Pulp	249ml	110	0	0	0	0	0	26
Tropicana Pure Premium Orange Juice with Calcium, Vitamin D & Lots of Pulp	249ml	110	0	0	0	0	0	26
Tropicana Pure Premium Orange Juice with Calcium, Vitamin D & Pulp	249g	110	0	0	0	0	0	26
Tropicana Pure Premium Orange Juice with Lots of Pulp	240ml	110	0	0	0	0	0	26
Tropicana Pure Premium Orange Juice with No Pulp	368ml	170	0	0	0	0	0	39
Tropicana Pure Premium Orange Juice with Some Pulp	240ml	110	0	0	0	0	0	26
Tropicana Pure Premium Orange Tangerine Juice	249g	110	0	0	0	0	0	25
Tropicana Pure Premium Ruby Red Grapefruit Juice	247g	90	0	0	0	0	0	22
Tropicana Pure Raspberry Acai Juice	246ml	140	1	0	0	0	15	30
Tropicana Pure Valencia Mango Juice	249ml	130	0	0	0	0	10	30
Tropicana Pure Valencia Orange Juice with Pulp	250ml	120	0	0	0	0	0	27
Tropicana Twister Orange Soda	361ml	190	0	0	0	0	35	52

Beverages

	Serving	Calories	Total fat (gm)	Saturated fat (gm)	Trans fats (gm)	Cholesterol (mg)	Sodium (mg)	Carbs (gm)
V8 Spicy Hot Vegetable Juice	240ml	50	0	0	0	0	620	10
V8 Splash Fruit Juice	248ml	70	0	0	0	0	50	18
V8 V Fusion Light Fruit Juice	250ml	50	0	0	0	0	40	13
V8 V Fusion Tropical Orange Juice	243ml	120	0	0	0	0	80	28
V8 Vegetable Juice	340ml	70	0	0	0	0	200	15
Vanilla Coke Zero	355ml	0	0	0	0	0	40	0
Vault Citrus Soda	355ml	180	0	0	0	0	45	47
Vernor's Ginger Ale	244ml	100	0	0	0	0	15	26
Welch's Concord Grape Juice	312ml	210	0	0	0	0	25	53
Welch's Juice Cocktail	253ml	140	0	0	0	0	5	34
Welch's White Grape Juice	250ml	160	0	0	0	0	20	39
Welch's White Grape Peach Juice	240ml	160	0	0	0	0	15	39
Welch's Grape Juice	253ml	180	0	0	0	0	20	45
Welch's Grape Soda	391ml	190	0	0	0	0	55	51
Wild Cherry Pepsi	240ml	100	0	0	0	0	20	28

Grocery Food Factoid:

Of the top 10 best selling foods 7 are soda. Here's the top 10 list:

1. Coke Classic
2. Diet Coke
3. Pepsi
4. Dr. Pepper
5. Mountain Dew
6. Diet Pepsi
7. Sprite
8. Kraft Philadelphia Cream Cheese
9. Lay's potato chips
10. Nabisco Oreo cookies

SHOPPING LIST/NOTES:

_____

_____

_____

_____

_____

_____

_____

Breakfast Foods

	Serving	Calories	Total fat (gm)	Saturated fat (gm)	Trans fats (gm)	Cholesterol (mg)	Sodium (mg)	Carbs (gm)
Aunt Jemima Buttermilk Pancake/Waffle Mix	45g	160	2	0.5	0	10	460	31
Aunt Jemima Original Pancake/Waffle Mix	46g	160	1.5	0	0	5	470	32
Bear Naked Fruit & Nut Granola	30g	140	7	1.5	0	0	0	18
Bear Naked Peak Protein Original Granola	30g	140	7	0.5	0	0	20	16
Bisquick Shake N' Pour Buttermilk Pancake Mix	63g	220	3	1	0.5	0	800	42
Cascadian Farm Honey & Oats Granola	55g	230	6	1	0	0	110	42
Cream of Wheat Hot Cereal	33g	120	0	0	0	0	0	24
Cream of Wheat Maple & Brown Sugar Hot Cereal	35g	130	0	0	0	0	140	28
Cream of Wheat Original Instant Hot Cereal	28g	100	0	0	0	0	160	19
General Mills Apple Cinnamon Cheerios	30g	120	1.5	0	0	0	120	25
General Mills Banana Nut Cheerios	28g	100	1	0	0	0	160	23
General Mills Basic 4 Multigrain Cereal	55g	200	2.5	0.5	0	0	320	43
General Mills Berry Burst Cheerios	27g	100	1	0	0	0	170	22
General Mills Cheerios	28g	100	2	0	0	0	190	20
General Mills Chocolate Chex	32g	130	2.5	0.5	0	0	230	26
General Mills Cinnamon Toast Crunch	31g	130	3	0.5	0	0	220	25
General Mills Cocoa Puffs	27g	110	1.5	0	0	0	150	23
General Mills Cookie Crisp Cereal	26g	100	1	0	0	0	150	22
General Mills Corn Chex	31g	120	0.5	0	0	0	290	26
General Mills Fiber One Caramel Delight Cereal	50g	180	3	0	0	0	260	41
General Mills Fiber One Cereal	30g	60	1	0	0	0	105	25
General Mills Fiber One Frosted Wheat	60g	200	1	0	0	0	0	49
General Mills Fiber One Honey Clusters Cereal	52g	160	1.5	0	0	0	280	42
General Mills Fiber One Raisin Bran	55g	170	1	0	0	0	260	45
General Mills Frosted Cheerios	28g	110	1	0	0	0	170	23
General Mills Fruity Cheerios	27g	100	1	0	0	0	135	23
General Mills Honey Nut Cheerios	28g	110	1.5	0	0	0	190	22
General Mills Honey Nut Chex	32g	120	0.5	0	0	0	230	28
General Mills Honey Nut Clusters	57g	210	1	0	0	0	290	49
General Mills Kix	30g	110	1	0	0	0	210	25
General Mills Lucky Charms	27g	110	1	0	0	0	190	22
General Mills Multi Bran Chex	47g	160	1.5	0	0	0	310	39
General Mills Multigrain Cheerios	29g	110	1	0	0	0	200	23
General Mills Oat Cluster Cheerios	27g	100	1	0	0	0	140	22
General Mills Oatmeal Crisp	60g	240	4.5	0.5	0	0	130	47
General Mills Raisin Nut Bran	49g	180	3	0.5	0	0	230	38

Breakfast Foods

Breakfast Foods	Serving	Calories	Total fat (gm)	Saturated fat (gm)	Trans fats (gm)	Cholesterol (mg)	Sodium (mg)	Carbs (gm)
General Mills Raisin Oatmeal Crisp	62g	230	2.5	0.5	0	0	135	51
General Mills Reese's Puffs Cereal	29g	120	3	0.5	0	0	180	22
General Mills Rice Chex	27g	100	0.5	0	0	0	240	23
General Mills Strawberry Chex	31g	130	2	0	0	0	200	26
General Mills Total	30g	100	0.5	0	0	0	190	23
General Mills Total Cinnamon Crunch	51g	190	2.5	0	0	0	200	40
General Mills Total Cranberry Crunch	58g	190	1.5	0	0	0	280	44
General Mills Total Raisin Bran	53g	160	1	0	0	0	250	40
General Mills Trix	32g	120	1.5	0	0	0	180	28
General Mills Wheat Chex	47g	160	1	0	0	0	340	38
General Mills Wheaties	27g	100	0.5	0	0	0	190	22
General Mills Yogurt Burst Cheerios	30g	120	1.5	0.5	0	0	180	24
General Mills Golden Grahams	31g	120	1	0	0	0	270	26
Hungry Jack Buttermilk Pancake/Waffle Mix	44g	150	1.5	0	0	5	550	31
Hungry Jack Pancake/Waffle Mix	44g	150	2	0	0	5	600	30
Kashi Heart To Heart Honey Toasted Oats	33g	110	1.5	0	0	0	90	25
Kashi Honey Sunshine 7 Whole Grain Cereal	30g	100	1.5	0	0	0	135	25
Kashi Organic Autumn Wheat Cereal	54g	190	1	0	0	0	0	45
Kashi Organic Cinnamon Harvest Cereal	54g	190	1	0	0	0	0	44
Kashi Organic Strawberry Fields Cereal	32g	120	0	0	0	0	200	28
Kashi Go Lean Crunch	53g	200	4.5	0	0	0	140	36
Kashi Go Lean Honey Multigrain Crunch with Soy Protein	52g	140	1	0	0	0	85	30
Kashi Go Lean Multigrain Crunch with Protein	53g	190	3	0	0	0	100	37
Kellogg's All Bran	31g	80	1	0	0	0	80	23
Kellogg's All Bran Bran Buds	30g	70	1	0	0	0	200	24
Kellogg's All Bran Complete	29g	90	0.5	0	0	0	210	23
Kellogg's All Bran Strawberry Medley	55g	170	1.5	0	0	0	230	44
Kellogg's Apple Jack's	28g	110	0.5	0	0	0	135	25
Kellogg's Cocoa Krispies Cereal Straws	31g	140	3.5	2	0	0	15	24
Kellogg's Cocoa Rice Krispies	31g	120	1	0.5	0	0	160	27
Kellogg's Corn Flakes	28g	100	0	0	0	0	200	24
Kellogg's Corn Pops	29g	0	0	0	0	0	110	26
Kellogg's Cracklin' Oat Bran	49g	200	7	3	0	0	150	35
Kellogg's Crispix	29g	110	0	0	0	0	210	25
Kellogg's Froot Loops	29g	110	1	0.5	0	0	135	25
Kellogg's Froot Loops Cereal Straws	31g	140	3.5	2	0	0	15	24
Kellogg's Frosted Flakes	30g	110	0	0	0	0	140	27

Breakfast Foods

Breakfast Foods	Serving	Calories	Total fat (gm)	Saturated fat (gm)	Trans fats (gm)	Cholesterol (mg)	Sodium (mg)	Carbs (gm)
Kellogg's Frosted Flakes with 1/3 Less Sugar	31g	120	0	0	0	0	180	28
Kellogg's Frosted Flakes Gold	31g	110	0.5	0	0	0	190	27
Kellogg's Frosted Mini Wheats	51g	180	1	0	0	0	5	41
Kellogg's Frosted Pop Tarts	52g	200	5	1.5	0	0	170	37
Kellogg's Fruit & Yogurt Special K	32g	120	1	0.5	0	0	135	27
Kellogg's Honey Smacks	27g	100	0.5	0	0	0	50	24
Kellogg's Keebler Cookie Crunch	30g	110	1	0	0	0	170	26
Kellogg's Little Bites Chocolate Mini Wheats	55g	200	2	1	0	0	200	45
Kellogg's Nutri-Grain Flavored Cereal Bars	37g	130	3	0.5	0	0	105	24
Kellogg's Pop Tarts, Unfrosted	52g	200	5	2	0	0	210	36
Kellogg's Product 19 Cereal	30g	100	0	0	0	0	210	25
Kellogg's Protein Plus Special K	29g	100	3	0.5	0	0	110	14
Kellogg's Raisin Bran	59g	190	1.5	0	0	0	350	45
Kellogg's Raisin Bran Crunch	53g	190	1	0	0	0	210	45
Kellogg's Raisin Bran Extra	56g	190	3	1.5	0	0	350	44
Kellogg's Rice Krispies	33g	120	0	0	0	0	320	29
Kellogg's Smart Start	50g	190	0.5	0	0	0	280	43
Kellogg's Smart Start Healthy Heart Cinnamon Raisin Oat Bran	51g	180	2	0.5	0	0	115	39
Kellogg's Smart Start Toasted Whole Grain Oats	60g	220	2.5	0.5	0	0	140	48
Kellogg's Special K	31g	120	0.5	0	0	0	220	22
Kellogg's Special K Blueberry Cereal Bars	23g	90	1.5	1	0	0	95	18
Kellogg's Special K Cinnamon Pecan Cereal Bars	22g	90	1.5	0	0	0	115	17
Kellogg's Special K Honey Nut Cereal Bars	22g	90	2	0	0	0	110	16
Kellogg's Special K Red Berries Cereal Straws	31g	110	0	0	0	0	220	25
Kellogg's Strawberry Smart Start	55g	200	2.5	0.5	0	0	130	43
Krusteaz Belgian Waffle Mix	79g	290	2.5	0.5	0	0	850	58
Krusteaz Blueberry Pancake Mix	66g	240	2.5	1	0	20	640	47
Krusteaz Buttermilk Pancake Mix	57g	210	2	0.5	0	5	560	42
Malt-O-Meal Cinnamon Toasters	30g	130	3.5	0.5	0	0	140	24
Malt-O-Meal Frosted Mini Spooners	55g	190	1	0	0	0	10	45
Malt-O-Meal Marshmallows Mateys	30g	120	1	0	0	0	200	25
Malt-O-Meal Scooters	30g	110	1.5	0	0	0	210	24
Malt-O-Meal Tootie Fruities	32g	130	1	0	0	0	150	28
Malt-O-Meal Golden Puffs	27g	110	0	0	0	0	65	24
Nature's Path Flax Plus Granola with Pumpkin Seeds	30g	140	5	1	0	0	25	20

Breakfast Foods

Breakfast Foods	Serving	Calories	Total fat (gm)	Saturated fat (gm)	Trans fats (gm)	Cholesterol (mg)	Sodium (mg)	Carbs (gm)
Nestle Carnation French Vanilla Instant Breakfast	36g	130	0	0	0	5	100	27
Nestle Carnation Milk Chocolate Instant Breakfast	20g	60	0.5	0	0	5	60	12
Nestle Hot Cocoa Mix	20g	80	3	2	0	0	160	15
Nestle Nesquik Chocolate Powder	16g	60	0.5	0	0	0	30	14
Ovaltine Chocolate Powder	21g	80	0	0	0	0	115	18
Post Bran Flakes	30g	100	0.5	0	0	0	220	24
Post Cocoa Pebbles	30g	110	1.5	1	0	0	180	26
Post Cranberry Vanilla Trail Mix Crunch	48g	190	4	0	0	0	135	36
Post Frosted Wheat	52g	180	1	0	0	0	0	43
Post Fruity Pebbles	30g	110	1	1	0	0	180	26
Post Honey Bunches of Oats	30g	120	2	0	0	0	150	25
Post Honey Nut Shredded Wheat	52g	190	1.5	0	0	0	70	44
Post Honeycomb Cereal	32g	130	1	0	0	0	180	28
Post Raisin & Almond Trail Mix Crunch	48g	180	2.5	0	0	0	210	37
Post Raisin Bran	59g	190	1	0	0	0	300	46
Post Selects Banana Nut Crunch	59g	240	6	0.5	0	0	230	44
Post Selects Blueberry Morning	55g	220	3	0	0	0	280	45
Post Selects Cranberry Almond Crunch	51g	200	3.5	0	0	0	115	39
Post Selects Great Grains with Pecans	51g	210	6	0.5	0	0	150	38
Post Selects Great Grains with Raisins, Dates & Pecans	54g	210	4.5	0	0	0	130	40
Post Shredded Wheat	47g	160	1	0	0	0	0	37
Post Spoon Size Shredded Wheat	49g	170	1	0	0	0	0	40
Post Waffle Crisps	30g	120	2.5	0	0	0	115	25
Post Golden Crisp	27g	110	0	0	0	0	25	24
Post Grape-Nuts	58g	200	1	0	0	0	290	48
Quaker 100% Natural Granola	48g	210	6	3.5	0	0	20	35
Quaker 100% Natural Granola with Raisins	51g	210	6	3.5	0	0	25	38
Quaker Butter Instant Grits	28g	100	1.5	0.5	0	0	340	21
Quaker Cap'N Crunch	27g	110	1.5	1	0	0	200	23
Quaker Cap'N Crunch Crunch Berries	26g	100	1.5	1	0	0	180	22
Quaker Cap'N Crunch Peanut Butter Crunch	27g	110	2.5	1	0	0	200	21
Quaker Cinnamon Life	32g	120	1.5	0	0	0	150	25
Quaker Cinnamon Oatmeal Squares	60g	230	2.5	0.5	0	0	260	48
Quaker Dinosaur Eggs Brown Sugar Oatmeal	50g	190	3.5	2	0	0	260	37
Quaker Flavored Instant Oatmeal	31g	110	1.5	0.4	0	0	170	3
Quaker Honey Graham Oh's	27g	110	2	1.5	0	0	170	23
Quaker Kretschmer Original Wheatgerm	13g	50	1	0	0	0	0	6

Breakfast Foods

Breakfast Foods	Serving	Calories	Total fat (gm)	Saturated fat (gm)	Trans fats (gm)	Cholesterol (mg)	Sodium (mg)	Carbs (gm)
Quaker Life	32g	80	1	0	0	0	110	16
Quaker Maple & Brown Sugar Life	32g	120	1.5	0	0	0	150	25
Quaker Oatmeal Chocolate Chip Breakfast Cookies	48g	180	6	2	0	5	190	31
Quaker Oatmeal Squares	56g	210	2.5	0.5	0	0	250	44
Quaker Oatmeal To Go Brown Sugar & Cinnamon Cereal Bars	60g	220	4	1	0	15	230	43
Quaker Old Fashioned Oats	40g	150	3	0.5	0	0	0	27
Quaker Original Oatmeal	28g	100	2	0	0	0	80	19
Quaker Quick Hominy Grits	37g	130	0.5	0	0	0	0	29
Quaker Quick Oats	40g	150	3	0.5	0	0	0	27
Quaker Simple Harvest Instant Oatmeal	42g	160	3.5	0.5	0	0	75	30
Quaker Weight Control Instant Oatmeal	45g	160	3	0.5	0	0	260	29
Stella Doro Breakfast Cookies	21g	90	3	1.5	0	20	65	14
Swiss Miss Hot Cocoa Mix	16g	60	1	1	0	0	170	10

Grocery Food Factoid:

In the world there are three populations that live longer, healthier lives than anyone else. These include Sicilians who eat a Mediterranean diet, Okinawans from Japan, and 7th Day Adventists. These people have longer life spans than any other groups in the world. They don't eat processed foods. You can avoid most processed foods by choosing foods that are green.

Grocery Food Factoid:

91% ... The percentage of all type II diabetes that is caused by a poor diet and lack of exercise. As we gain weight, we are more likely to become diabetic. In many states 1 in 10 adults is diabetic.

SHOPPING LIST/NOTES:

_____
_____
_____
_____
_____
_____
_____
_____
_____

Canned Goods

	Serving	Calories	Total fat (gm)	Saturated fat (gm)	Trans fats (gm)	Cholesterol (mg)	Sodium (mg)	Carbs (gm)
B&M Original Baked Beans	131g	160	1	0.2	0	5	390	31
Bruce's Sweet Yams	166g	150	0.5	0	0	0	45	36
Bush's Best Baked Beans	130g	150	1	0	0	0	440	31
Bush's Best Black Beans	130g	105	0.5	0	0	0	480	23
Bush's Best Honey Baked Beans	130g	160	1	0	0	0	540	32
Bush's Best Kidney Beans	130g	100	0	0	0	0	260	22
Bush's Best Maple Cured Bacon Baked Beans	130g	140	1	0	0	0	620	28
Bush's Best Onion Baked Beans	130g	140	1	0	0	0	550	29
Bush's Best Original Baked Beans	130g	140	1	0	0	0	550	29
Bush's Best Pinto Beans	130g	80	0	0	0	0	450	18
Bush's Best Seasoned Black Beans	130g	110	0.5	0	0	0	450	23
Bush's Best Vegetarian Baked Beans	130g	130	0	0	0	0	550	29
Bush's Best Garbanzo Beans	130g	105	2	0	0	0	470	20
Bush's Best Great Northern Beans	130g	80	0	0	0	0	460	17
Bush's Best Grillin' Baked Beans	130g	170	0.5	0	0	0	480	35
Campbell's Beef Gravy	59ml	25	1	0.5	0	5	270	3
Campbell's Chicken Gravy	59ml	40	3	1	0	5	260	3
Campbell's Pork & Beans	130g	140	1.5	0.5	0	5	440	25
Campbell's Turkey Gravy	59ml	25	1	0.5	0	5	270	3
Contadina Italian Tomato Paste	33g	35	0.5	0	0	0	290	7
Contadina Tomato Paste No Additives	33g	30	0	0	0	0	20	6
Contadina Tomato Sauce No Additives	61g	15	0	0	0	0	280	3
Del Monte Citrus Fruit	113g	40	0	0	0	0	10	12
Del Monte Diced Pears in Light Syrup	113g	70	0	0	0	0	10	18
Del Monte Fresh Cut Carrots	123g	35	0	0	0	0	300	8
Del Monte Fresh Cut Corn	125g	60	0.5	0	0	0	360	14
Del Monte Fresh Cut French Green Beans	121g	20	0	0	0	0	390	4
Del Monte Fresh Cut French Green Beans No Salt Added	121g	20	0	0	0	0	10	4
Del Monte Fresh Cut Lima Beans	126g	80	0	0	0	0	390	15
Del Monte Fresh Cut No Salt Added Corn	125g	60	1	0	0	0	10	11
Del Monte Fresh Cut No Salt Added Creamed Corn	125g	60	0.5	0	0	0	10	14
Del Monte Fresh Cut Specialties Whole Green Beans	121g	20	0	0	0	0	390	4
Del Monte Fresh Cut Spinach	115g	30	0	0	0	0	360	4
Del Monte Fresh Cut Summer Crisp Corn	105g	70	1	0	0	0	270	13
Del Monte Fresh Cut Sweet Corn	125g	60	1	0	0	0	360	11
Del Monte Fresh Cut Sweet Peas	125g	60	0	0	0	0	390	13

Canned Goods

Canned Goods	Serving	Calories	Total fat (gm)	Saturated fat (gm)	Trans fats (gm)	Cholesterol (mg)	Sodium (mg)	Carbs (gm)
Del Monte Fresh Cut Sweet Peas No Salt Added	125g	60	0	0	0	0	10	11
Del Monte Fresh Cut Green Beans	121g	20	0	0	0	0	390	4
Del Monte Fresh Cut Green Beans No Salt Added	121g	20	0	0	0	0	10	4
Del Monte Fruit Cocktail	127g	100	0	0	0	0	10	24
Del Monte Fruit To Go Citrus Fruit	113g	70	0	0	0	0	10	17
Del Monte Fruit To Go Wildberry Diced Mixed Fruit	113g	70	0	0	0	0	10	18
Del Monte Lite Pear Halves in Extra Light Syrup	124g	60	0	0	0	0	10	15
Del Monte Mild Green Chilies & Diced Tomatoes	126g	30	0	0	0	0	450	6
Del Monte Mixed Fruit	113g	70	0	0	0	0	10	18
Del Monte Onion, Celery & Green Pepper Tomatoes	126g	35	0	0	0	0	360	9
Del Monte Sliced Pears	127g	100	0	0	0	0	10	24
Del Monte Tomatoes	126g	25	0	0	0	0	200	6
Del Monte Very Cherry Mixed Fruit	124g	90	0	0	0	0	10	22
Del Monte Yellow Cling Peaches in Extra Light Syrup	124g	60	0	0	0	0	10	15
Del Monte Yellow Cling Peaches in Fruit Juice	124g	60	0	0	0	0	10	15
Del Monte Yellow Cling Peaches in Heavy Syrup	127g	100	0	0	0	0	10	24
Del Monte Yellow Cling Peaches in Light Syrup	113g	70	0	0	0	0	10	17
Del Monte Yellow Cling Peaches in Water	121g	30	0	0	0	0	10	7
Del Monte Garlic Oregano & Basil Tomatoes	126g	35	0	0	0	0	360	8
Dole Apple Parfait	123g	120	2	1	0	0	10	25
Dole Citrus Fruit	122g	80	0	0	0	0	5	21
Dole Diced Pears in Light Syrup	113g	80	0	0	0	0	0	19
Dole Fruit Bowls Cherry Mixed Fruit	113g	80	0	0	0	0	10	19
Dole Fruit Bowls Citrus Fruit in Orange Gel	123g	80	0	0	0	0	25	23
Dole Fruit Bowls Mandarin Oranges in Light Syrup	113g	70	0	0	0	0	10	18
Dole Fruit Bowls No Sugar Added Pineapple in Pineapple Juice	113g	60	0	0	0	0	10	16
Dole Fruit Bowls Peaches in Strawberry Gel	123g	90	0	0	0	0	25	23
Dole Fruit Bowls Pineapple in Lime Gel	123g	80	0	0	0	0	80	21
Dole Fruit Bowls Yellow Cling Diced Peaches in Light Syrup	113g	80	0	0	0	0	15	19
Dole Mixed Fruit	113g	80	0	0	0	0	0	19
Dole Mixed Fruit in Black Cherry Gel	123g	100	0	0	0	0	25	24

Canned Goods

	Serving	Calories	Total fat (gm)	Saturated fat (gm)	Trans fats (gm)	Cholesterol (mg)	Sodium (mg)	Carbs (gm)
Dole No Sugar Added Pineapple in Pineapple Juice	122g	70	0	0	0	0	10	15
Dole Peach Parfait in Water	123g	120	2	2	0	0	10	24
Dole Pineapple in Heavy Syrup	123g	90	0	0	0	0	10	24
Dole Pineapple in Light Syrup	122g	80	0	0	0	0	0	21
Dole Pineapple in Pineapple Juice	122g	70	0	0	0	0	10	17
Dole Tropical Fruit Salad	122g	90	0	0	0	0	0	21
Dole Tropical Mixed Fruit in Light Syrup	122g	80	0	0	0	0	0	21
Dole Yellow Cling Peaches in Light Syrup	122g	80	0	0	0	0	0	21
El Pato Mexican Tomato Sauce	28g	5	0	0	0	0	135	1
Glory Foods Collard Greens	118g	35	0	0	0	0	490	5
Glory Foods Seasoned Mixed Greens	118g	35	0	0	0	0	490	4
Goya Black Beans	122g	90	0.5	0	0	0	460	19
Goya Spanish Tomato Sauce No Additives	61g	20	0	0	0	0	280	4
Goya Whole Pigeon Peas	125g	70	0	0	0	0	390	14
Green Giant Corn	124g	80	0.5	0	0	0	360	18
Green Giant 50% Less Sodium Corn	121g	80	0.5	0	0	0	180	16
Green Giant Asparagus Spears	126g	20	0	0	0	0	430	3
Green Giant Cream Sweet Corn	127g	90	0.5	0	0	0	400	19
Green Giant French Green Beans	118g	20	0	0	0	0	390	4
Green Giant Mexicorn Zesty Corn & Pepper	78g	70	0.5	0	0	0	250	14
Green Giant Mushrooms	68g	25	0	0	0	0	440	4
Green Giant Young Peas	122g	60	0	0	0	0	400	12
Green Giant Green Beans	120g	20	0	0	0	0	400	4
Hunt's Basil, Garlic & Oregano Tomato Sauce	62g	15	0	0	0	0	360	3
Hunt's Fire Roasted Tomatoes	123g	30	0	0	0	0	340	6
Hunt's Tomato Paste No Additives	33g	25	0	0	0	0	105	6
Hunt's Tomato Sauce No Additives	62g	20	0	0	0	0	20	5
Hunt's Tomatoes	121g	25	0	0	0	0	310	6
Hunt's Tomatoes No Additives	121g	40	0	0	0	0	290	8
Hunt's Garlic, Oregano & Basil Tomatoes	121g	35	0	0	0	0	370	7
Juanita's Mexican Hominy	130g	60	0.5	0	0	0	190	10
Le Sueur Very Young Early Peas	121g	60	0	0	0	0	380	12
Mott's Cinnamon Applesauce	128g	120	0	0	0	0	0	29
Mott's Healthy Harvest Granny Smith Applesauce	111g	50	0	0	0	0	0	13
Mott's Natural Applesauce	123g	50	0	0	0	0	0	14
Mott's Original Applesauce	128g	110	0	0	0	0	0	27
Mott's Strawberry Applesauce	113g	90	0	0	0	0	0	23

Canned Goods

Canned Goods	Serving	Calories	Total fat (gm)	Saturated fat (gm)	Trans fats (gm)	Cholesterol (mg)	Sodium (mg)	Carbs (gm)
Ocean Spray Whole Cranberry Sauce	70g	110	0	0	0	0	10	25
Princella Sweet Yams	162g	160	0	0	0	0	35	37
Ranch Style Western Pinto Beans	131g	130	2.5	1	0	0	590	20
Randall Great Northern Beans	113g	100	0	0	0	0	400	19
Red Pack Crushed Tomatoes	61g	20	0	0	0	0	120	4
Reese Quartered Artichoke Hearts	130g	50	0	0	0	0	380	9
Rotel Chili Pepper & Jalapeno Pepper Tomatoes	125g	20	0	0	0	0	520	4
Rotel Lime Juice & Cilantro Tomatoes	125g	30	0	0	0	0	540	6
Rotel Green Chile Tomatoes	125g	20	0	0	0	0	520	4
Tuttorosso Basil Tomatoes	61g	20	0	0	0	0	210	4
Van Camps' Beanee Weenee Original Beans & Wieners	220g	240	8	3	0	40	990	29
Van Camp's Pork & Beans	130g	110	1	0	0	0	390	23

Grocery Food Factoid:
Of the 14 different grocery food categories in this guide, produce is obviously the healthiest. Do you know which categories have the most unhealthy foods?
Baking Items and Packaged Desserts

Grocery Food Factoid:
There are over 3,500 foods in this guide. The ones with the most cholesterol are all products from Jimmy Dean. The top Jimmy Dean Sausage products have over 350mg of cholesterol per serving.

SHOPPING LIST/NOTES:
_____
_____
_____
_____
_____
_____
_____
_____
_____
_____
_____
_____

Condiments & Sauces

	Serving	Calories	Total fat (gm)	Saturated fat (gm)	Trans fats (gm)	Cholesterol (mg)	Sodium (mg)	Carbs (gm)
A-1 Steak Sauce	17g	15	0	0	0	0	280	3
Aunt Jemima Butter Pancake/Waffles Syrup	79ml	210	0	0	0	0	210	53
Aunt Jemima Lite Butter Pancake/Waffles Syrup with 30% Less Sugar	60ml	100	0	0	0	0	210	26
Aunt Jemima Lite Pancake/Waffles Syrup with 30% Less Sugar	60ml	100	0	0	0	0	190	26
Aunt Jemima Original Pancake/Waffles Syrup	79ml	210	0	0	0	0	120	52
Aunt Nellie's Pickled Beets	29g	15	0	0	0	0	55	4
Barilla Mushroom & Garlic Pasta Sauce	125g	70	2	0	0	0	450	12
Barilla Olive Oil Marinara Pasta Sauce	125g	70	1.5	0	0	0	460	12
Barilla Roasted Garlic Pasta Sauce	125g	60	1	0	0	0	460	12
Barilla Tomato & Basil Pasta Sauce	125g	60	1	0	0	0	460	12
Bertolli Olive Oil & Garlic Pasta Sauce	127g	90	3	0	0	0	500	14
Bertolli Parmesan Cheese Alfredo Pasta Sauce	61g	110	10	5	0	40	460	3
Bertolli Portobello Mushroom Alfredo Pasta Sauce	61g	80	6	3	0	30	420	3
Bertolli Vineyard Premium Collections Burgundy Wine Marinara Pasta Sauce	126g	80	2	0	0	0	500	14
Bertolli Vodka Pasta Sauce	125g	150	9	4.5	0	25	730	12
Bertolli Garlic Alfredo Pasta Sauce	61g	110	10	4	0	30	360	3
Black Pearls Olives	16g	25	2	0	0	0	95	1
Bob's Red Mill Flaxseed Seasoning	13g	60	4.5	0	0	0	0	4
Bonne Maman Strawberry Preserves	20g	50	0	0	0	0	0	13
Brianna's Rich Poppy Seed Salad Dressing	30ml	160	14	1	0	0	220	7
Buitoni Alfredo Pasta Sauce	61g	140	12	7	0.5	30	380	4
Buitoni Marinara Marinade	125g	70	3	0.5	0	0	560	10
Buitoni Pesto Pasta Sauce	62g	300	28	5	0	20	540	6
Bull's Eye Original Barbecue Sauce	30ml	50	0	0	0	0	310	13
Carroll Shelby's Original Texas Chili Seasoning Mix	19g	60	1	0	0	0	1320	12
Chi-Chi's Mild Salsa	30g	10	0	0	0	0	150	2
Cholula Mexican Hot Sauce	5g	0	0	0	0	0	85	0
Classico Creations Basil Pesto Pasta Sauce	62g	230	21	3	0	0	720	6
Classico Signature Recipes Alfredo Pasta Sauce	60g	100	9	5	0	50	410	3
Classico Signature Recipes Cabernet Marinara Pasta Sauce	125g	70	1.5	0	0	0	330	11
Classico Signature Recipes Caramel Onion & Roasted Garlic Pasta Sauce	125g	85	2.5	0.5	0	0	510	13
Classico Signature Recipes Fire Roasted Tomato Pasta Sauce	125g	50	0.5	0	0	0	320	10

Condiments & Sauces

	Serving	Calories	Total fat (gm)	Saturated fat (gm)	Trans fats (gm)	Cholesterol (mg)	Sodium (mg)	Carbs (gm)
Classico Signature Recipes Roasted Red Pepper Alfredo Pasta Sauce	60g	60	5	3	0	35	310	3
Classico Signature Recipes Roasted Garlic Alfredo Pasta Sauce	60g	70	6	3	0	30	430	3
Classico Signature Recipes Spicy Red Pepper Pasta Sauce	125g	60	2.5	0.5	0	0	300	8
Classico Signature Recipes Sun Dried Tomato Alfredo Pasta Sauce	60g	90	7	4	0	35	430	4
Classico Signature Recipes Tomato & Basil Pasta Sauce	125g	70	2	0	0	0	420	10
Classico Signature Recipes Vodka Pasta Sauce	125g	120	7	3	0	15	490	12
Classico Traditional Favorites Basil Pasta Sauce	125g	70	1	0	0	0	520	13
Classico Traditional Favorites Four Cheese Pasta Sauce	125g	90	3.5	1	0	0	490	11
Classico Traditional Favorites Italian Sausage Pasta Sauce	125g	80	2.5	1	0	5	430	10
Classico Traditional Favorites Roasted Garlic Pasta Sauce	125g	60	1	0	0	0	220	11
Classico Traditional Favorites Tomato & Basil Pasta Sauce	125g	50	1	0	0	0	380	9
Claussen Dill Pickles	28g	5	0	0	0	0	330	1
Claussen Hearty Garlic Dill Pickles	34g	5	0	0	0	0	320	1
Dale's All Purpose Marinade	18g	15	0	0	0	0	1220	1
Dean's French Onion Dip	30g	60	5	2.5	0	0	170	2
Dean's Liquid Half & Half	30ml	40	3	2	0	15	15	1
Dean's Guacamole Dip	30g	90	9	2.5	0	5	170	2
Del Monte Traditional Spaghetti Sauce	125g	70	1	0	0	0	590	14
Early California Black Thrown Olives	15g	25	2.5	0	0	0	115	1
Francesco Rinaldi Meat Pasta Sauce	125g	80	3.5	1	0	5	640	13
Francesco Rinaldi Original Pasta Sauce	125g	90	3	0.5	0	0	650	14
Francesco Rinaldi Tomato & Basil Pasta Sauce	125g	80	2.5	0	0	0	640	13
Francesco Rinaldi Tomato, Garlic & Onion Pasta Sauce	125g	80	2.5	0	0	0	640	13
Frank's Original Cayenne Pepper Hot Sauce	5ml	0	0	0	0	0	200	0
French's Original French Fried Onions	7g	45	3.5	1.5	0	0	60	3
French's Worcestershire Sauce	6ml	5	0	0	0	0	65	1
French's Yellow Honey Mustard	5g	10	0	0	0	0	30	1
French's Yellow Mustard	5g	0	0	0	0	0	55	0
Frito's Chili Cheese Dip	34g	45	3	1	0	0	290	3
Goober Creamy Peanut Butter Combo	53g	240	13	2.5	0	0	140	24
Good Seasons Italian Salad Dressing Mix	3g	5	0	0	0	0	320	1

Condiments & Sauces

	Serving	Calories	Total fat (gm)	Saturated fat (gm)	Trans fats (gm)	Cholesterol (mg)	Sodium (mg)	Carbs (gm)
Grandma's Mild Unsulphured Molasses	21ml	60	0	0	0	0	15	15
Heinz Beef Gravy	60g	30	1	0.5	0	5	390	4
Heinz Chili Sauce	17g	20	0	0	0	0	230	5
Heinz Cocktail Seafood Sauce	60g	60	0	0	0	0	690	15
Heinz Mushroom Gravy	60g	20	0.5	0	0	0	320	3
Heinz Pork Gravy	60g	20	0.5	0	0	0	350	3
Heinz Roasted Turkey Gravy	60g	25	1	0	0	5	290	3
Heinz Tomato Ketchup	17g	15	0	0	0	0	190	4
Heinz 57 Steak Sauce	17g	20	0	0	0	0	190	4
Hellmann's Light Mayonnaise	15g	35	3.5	0.5	0	5	130	1
Hellmann's Low Fat Mayonnaise	15g	15	1	0	0	0	130	2
Hellmann's Low Saturated Fat, Cholesterol Free Mayonnaise	13g	45	4.5	0	0	0	95	1
Hellmann's Mayonnaise	13g	90	10	1.5	0	5	90	0
Heluva Good French Onion Dip	31g	60	5	3	0	20	170	2
Hershey's Chocolate Syrup	39g	100	0	0	0	0	15	24
Hershey's Hot Fudge Ice Cream Syrup	37g	120	4	4	0	0	95	20
Hershey's Strawberry Syrup	40g	100	0	0	0	0	10	26
Hidden Valley Ranch Buttermilk Ranch Salad Dressing	30g	140	14	2	0	10	340	2
Hidden Valley Ranch Buttermilk Ranch Salad Dressing Mix	1g	0	0	0	0	0	140	1
Hidden Valley Ranch Fat Free Original Ranch Salad Dressing	32g	30	0	0	0	0	310	6
Hidden Valley Ranch Original Ranch Dip Mix	2g	5	0	0	0	0	240	1
Hidden Valley Ranch Original Ranch Salad Dressing	30ml	140	14	2.5	0	10	260	2
Hidden Valley Ranch Original Ranch Salad Dressing 50% Less Fat	31g	80	7	1	0	5	290	3
Hidden Valley Ranch Original Ranch Salad Dressing Mix	2g	5	0	0	0	0	135	1
Hormel Bacon Bits	7g	25	1.5	1	0	5	240	0
Hungry Jack Pancake/Waffle Syrup	79ml	210	0	0	0	0	140	53
Hunt's Four Cheese Spaghetti Sauce	126g	50	1	0	0	0	580	10
Hunt's Meat Spaghetti Sauce	126g	60	1	0	0	0	610	11
Hunt's Mushroom Spaghetti Sauce	126g	45	0.5	0	0	0	590	10
Hunt's Roasted Garlic & Onion Spaghetti Sauce	126g	50	1	0	0	0	540	10
Hunt's Tomato Ketchup	17g	20	0	0	0	0	190	4
Hunt's Traditional Spaghetti Sauce	126g	50	1	0	0	0	580	10
Hunt's Zesty & Spicy Spaghetti Sauce	126g	60	2	0	0	0	700	10
Hunt's Garlic & Herb Spaghetti Sauce	125g	40	1	0	0	0	610	8

Condiments & Sauces

	Serving	Calories	Total fat (gm)	Saturated fat (gm)	Trans fats (gm)	Cholesterol (mg)	Sodium (mg)	Carbs (gm)
International Delight Liquid Coffee Creamer	15ml	30	0	0	0	0	5	7
Jack Daniel's Original Barbecue Sauce	34g	50	0	0	0	0	290	12
Jif Creamy Peanut Butter	36g	190	12	2.5	0	0	250	15
Jif Crunchy Peanut Spread	36g	190	12	2.5	0	0	220	15
Jif Extra Crunchy Peanut Butter	32g	190	16	3	0	0	130	7
Karo Dark Corn Syrup	41ml	120	0	0	0	0	45	31
Karo Light Corn Syrup	30ml	120	0	0	0	0	30	30
KC Masterpiece Honey Teriyaki Marinade	15ml	40	0.5	0	0	0	360	9
KC Masterpiece Original Barbecue Sauce	36g	60	0	0	0	0	240	15
Kellogg's Eggo Buttery Pancake/Waffle Syrup	60ml	160	0	0	0	0	90	41
Kellogg's Eggo Original Pancake/Waffle Syrup	79ml	240	0	0	0	0	35	60
Ken's Steak House 50% Less Fat Raspberry Walnut Vinaigrette Salad Dressing	32g	80	6	1	0	0	125	7
Ken's Steak House 60% Less Fat Italian Salad Dressing	30g	50	5	1	0	0	330	1
Ken's Steak House 66% Less Fat Caesar Salad Dressing	31g	70	6	1	0	0	620	3
Ken's Steak House Blue Cheese Salad Dressing	30g	150	16	2.5	0	0	320	1
Ken's Steak House Buttermilk Ranch Salad Dressing	30g	180	20	3	0	5	280	1
Ken's Steak House Creamy Caesar Salad Dressing	29g	160	18	3	0	10	280	0
Ken's Steak House Honey Mustard Salad Dressing	30g	130	11	1.5	0	15	210	7
Ken's Steak House Ranch Salad Dressing	30g	140	15	2	0	10	310	2
Kikkoman Oriental Stir Fry Sauce	18g	20	0	0	0	0	520	4
Kitchen Bouquet Browning & Cooking Sauce	6g	15	0	0	0	0	10	3
Knorr Hollandaise Sauce Mix	14g	60	2.5	1	0	5	650	7
Kraft Catalina Salad Dressing	31g	130	11	1.5	0	0	380	7
Kraft Cheez Whiz Original Dip	33g	90	7	1.5	0	5	440	4
Kraft Creamy French Salad Dressing	31g	150	14	2	0	0	260	5
Kraft Free Catalina Salad Dressing	35g	50	0	0	0	0	350	11
Kraft Free Ranch Salad Dressing	34g	50	0	0	0	0	330	11
Kraft Free Thousand Island Salad Dressing	33g	45	0	0	0	0	260	10
Kraft French Onion Dip	31g	60	4.5	3	0	0	220	3
Kraft Hickory Smoked Barbecue Sauce	35g	50	0	0	0	0	430	12
Kraft Honey Barbecue Sauce	36g	50	0	0	0	0	360	13
Kraft Light 50% Less Fat Balsamic Vinaigrette Salad Dressing	31g	25	1	0	0	0	290	4

Condiments & Sauces

	Serving	Calories	Total fat (gm)	Saturated fat (gm)	Trans fats (gm)	Cholesterol (mg)	Sodium (mg)	Carbs (gm)
Kraft Light Done Right Ranch Salad Dressing	32g	80	6	1	0	10	440	7
Kraft Light Done Right Raspberry Vinaigrette with Virgin Olive Oil Salad Dressing	32g	60	4	0	0	0	270	5
Kraft Light Done Right Zesty Italian with Virgin Olive Oil Salad Dressing	31g	25	1.5	0	0	0	470	3
Kraft Mayo Light Mayonnaise	15g	45	4	0.5	0	5	95	2
Kraft Mayo Mayonnaise	15g	45	4	0	0	5	95	2
Kraft Mayonnaise	13g	90	10	1.5	0	5	70	0
Kraft Miracle Whip 50% Less Fat Salad Dressing	16g	20	1.5	0	0	5	135	2
Kraft Miracle Whip Salad Dressing	15g	35	3	0	0	0	100	2
Kraft Original Barbecue Sauce	36g	50	0	0	0	0	440	12
Kraft Original Tartar Sauce	31g	60	4.5	0.5	0	5	210	4
Kraft Ranch with Bacon Salad Dressing	29g	150	16	2.5	0	10	300	2
Kraft Ranchers Choice Ranch Salad Dressing	30g	120	12	2	0	0	370	3
Kraft Roka Blue Cheese Salad Dressing	29g	120	13	2	0	5	380	1
Kraft Special Collections Roasted Red Pepper Italian Salad Dressing	31g	40	2	0	0	0	440	4
Kraft Thick 'N Spicy Original Barbecue Sauce	35g	50	0	0	0	0	430	12
Kraft Thousand Island Salad Dressing	32g	110	10	1.5	0	5	330	5
Kraft Tuscan House Italian Salad Dressing	31g	130	13	1.5	0	5	250	3
Kraft Zesty Italian Salad Dressing	31g	70	6	0	0	0	370	3
La Costena Jalapeno Peppers	35g	5	0	0	0	0	580	1
Land O' Lakes Fat Free Half & Half	30ml	20	0	0	0	0	30	3
Land O' Lakes Half & Half	30ml	40	3	2	0	15	30	1
Land O' Lakes Low Fat Half & Half	30ml	25	1.5	1	0	5	15	1
Las Palmas Mild Enchilada Sauce	60g	15	0.5	0	0	0	310	2
Lawry's Teriyaki Fish & Chicken Meat Marinade	18ml	20	0	0	0	0	560	5
Lay's Creamy Ranch Dip	33g	60	5	2.5	0	5	240	1
Lea & Perrin's Original Worcestershire Sauce	5ml	5	0	0	0	0	65	1
Litehouse Chunky Bleu Cheese Salad Dressing	30ml	150	16	1.5	0	15	220	1
Log Cabin Lite Pancake/Waffle Syrup	60ml	120	0	0	0	0	150	30
Marie's Chunky Blue Cheese Salad Dressing	28g	160	17	3.5	0	15	170	0
Marie's Coleslaw Dressing	28g	150	13	2	0	10	170	8
Marie's Creamy Ranch Salad Dressing	28g	170	19	3	0	15	150	1
Mccormick Chili Seasoning Mix	9g	30	0.5	0	0	0	310	5

Condiments & Sauces

	Serving	Calories	Total fat (gm)	Saturated fat (gm)	Trans fats (gm)	Cholesterol (mg)	Sodium (mg)	Carbs (gm)
McCormick Meatloaf Seasoning Mix	4g	15	0	0	0	0	350	2
McCormick Sloppy Joe Seasoning Mix	5g	20	0	0	0	0	300	3
McCormick Taco Seasoning Mix	6g	20	0	0	0	0	430	3
McIllhenny Tabasco Pepper Hot Sauce	5ml	0	0	0	0	0	30	0
Mrs. Butterworth's Lite Pancake/Waffle Syrup	60ml	100	0	0	0	0	130	25
Mrs. Butterworth's Original Pancake/Waffle Syrup	79ml	210	0	0	0	0	115	53
Mrs. Butterworth's Sugar Free Low Calorie Pancake/Waffle Syrup	60ml	35	0	0	0	0	100	12
Mt. Olive's Dill Pickles	1 item	10	0	0	0	0	430	2
Nestle Coffee Mate 50% Less Fat Powder Coffee Creamer	2g	10	0	0	0	0	0	2
Nestle Coffee Mate Carb Select Liquid Coffee Creamer	15ml	15	1	0	0	0	5	1
Nestle Coffee Mate Liquid Coffee Creamer	15ml	35	1.5	0	0	0	10	5
Nestle Coffee Mate Original Fat Free Powder Coffee Creamer	2g	10	0	0	0	0	0	2
Nestle Nesquik Chocolate Dessert Syrup	38g	100	0	0	0	0	55	25
Newman's Own All Natural Marinara Pasta Sauce	125g	70	2	0	0	0	510	12
Newman's Own Balsamic Vinaigrette Salad Dressing	30g	90	9	1	0	0	350	3
Newman's Own Bombolina Tomato & Basil Pasta Sauce	125g	90	4.5	0.5	0	0	620	13
Newman's Own Italian Salad Dressing	30g	120	13	1	0	0	400	1
Newman's Own Lighten Up Balsamic Vinaigrette Salad Dressing	30g	45	4	0.5	0	0	470	2
Newman's Own Lighten Up Honey Mustard Salad Dressing	30g	70	4	0.5	0	0	290	7
Newman's Own Medium Salsa	32g	10	0	0	0	0	105	2
Newman's Own Olive Oil & Vinegar Salad Dressing	27g	150	16	2.5	0	0	150	1
Newman's Own Sockarooni Tomato, Pepper & Spices Pasta Sauce	124g	70	2	0	0	0	520	12
Old El Paso Chili Peppers	30g	10	0	0	0	0	120	2
Old El Paso Mild Enchilada Sauce	60g	25	1	0	0	0	260	3
Old El Paso Taco Seasoning Mix	5g	15	0	0	0	0	370	3
Open Pit Original Barbecue Sauce	34g	45	0	0	0	0	510	10
Organic Valley Liquid Half & Half	30ml	40	3.5	2	0	10	10	1
Ortega Chili Pepper	25g	5	0	0	0	0	70	1
Ortega Taco Sauce	16g	10	0	0	0	0	120	2
Ortega Taco Seasoning Mix	6g	20	0	0	0	0	430	4
Pace Picante Sauce	32ml	10	0	0	0	0	250	2

Condiments & Sauces

	Serving	Calories	Total fat (gm)	Saturated fat (gm)	Trans fats (gm)	Cholesterol (mg)	Sodium (mg)	Carbs (gm)
Pace Salsa	30ml	10	0	0	0	0	240	2
Peter Pan Creamy Peanut Butter	32g	190	17	3.5	0	0	140	6
Peter Pan Crunchy Peanut Butter	32g	190	16	3	0	0	110	6
Prego 3 Cheese Spaghetti Sauce	120ml	80	1.5	0.5	0	5	430	14
Prego Heart Smart Traditional Pasta Sauce	120ml	100	3	0.5	0	0	430	15
Prego Italian Sausage & Garlic Spaghetti Sauce	120ml	100	4	1	0	5	500	13
Prego Meat Spaghetti Sauce	120ml	100	4	1	0	5	580	13
Prego Mushroom & Garlic Pasta Sauce	120ml	80	2.5	0.5	0	0	470	13
Prego Mushroom Spaghetti Sauce	120ml	90	3	1	0	0	550	14
Prego Roasted Garlic & Herb Spaghetti Sauce	120ml	90	3.5	0.5	0	0	560	13
Prego Tomato, Basil & Garlic Pasta Sauce	120ml	80	2.5	0.5	0	0	420	12
Prego Tomato, Garlic & Onion Spaghetti Sauce	120ml	90	3	0.5	0	0	470	13
Prego Traditional Spaghetti Sauce	125ml	80	3	0	0	0	580	13
Prego Garden Combo Spaghetti Sauce	120ml	70	1.5	0.5	0	0	470	13
Ragu Alfredo Pasta Sauce	61g	110	10	3.5	0	30	350	2
Ragu Cheese Creations Parmesan Alfredo Pasta Sauce	61g	70	5	3	0	25	320	2
Ragu Double Cheddar Pasta Sauce	64g	100	9	3	0	25	450	3
Ragu Mushroom Pasta Sauce	128g	80	2.5	0	0	0	620	13
Ragu Old World Style Meat Pasta Sauce	125g	70	3	0.5	0	0	460	9
Ragu Old World Style Mushroom Pasta Sauce	125g	70	2.5	0	0	0	580	10
Ragu Old World Style Traditional Pasta Sauce	125g	70	2.5	0	0	0	480	10
Ragu Roasted Garlic Parmesan Pasta Sauce	64g	110	10	3	0	25	350	3
Ragu Robusto 7 Herb Tomato Pasta Sauce	129g	80	3	0	0	0	550	12
Ragu Robusto Parmesan Romano Pasta Sauce	129g	90	3	0.5	0	5	580	12
Ragu Robusto Roasted Garlic Pasta Sauce	129g	80	2.5	0	0	0	550	13
Ragu Robusto Sauteed Onion & Garlic Pasta Sauce	129g	90	3.5	0.5	0	0	550	12
Ragu Robusto Six Cheese Pasta Sauce	129g	90	3	1	0	5	580	12
Ragu Tomato Garlic Onion Pasta Sauce	128g	80	2.5	0	0	0	510	13
Ragu Traditional Pasta Sauce	125g	80	3	0	0	0	510	11
Ragu Garden Combination Pasta Sauce	128g	80	2.5	0	0	0	530	12
Ragu Green Pepper & Mushroom Pasta Sauce	128g	80	2.5	0	0	0	560	12
Raos Homemade All Natural Marinara Pasta Sauce	113g	70	4.5	0.5	0	0	350	6
Reese's Creamy Peanut Butter	32g	200	15	2	0	0	140	8

Condiments & Sauces

	Serving	Calories	Total fat (gm)	Saturated fat (gm)	Trans fats (gm)	Cholesterol (mg)	Sodium (mg)	Carbs (gm)
Sabra Hummus	28g	70	6	1	0	0	130	3
Sabra Roasted Red Pepper Hummus Spread	28g	70	6	1	0	0	120	3
Sabra Spicy Hummus	28g	80	6	0.5	0	0	150	4
Silk French Vanilla Liquid Coffee Creamer	15ml	20	1	0	0	0	10	3
Simply Jif Creamy Peanut Butter	31g	190	16	3	0	0	65	6
Skippy Creamy Peanut Butter	32g	190	16	3	0	0	150	7
Skippy Honey Nut Creamy Peanut Butter	32g	190	16	0	0	0	125	7
Skippy Natural Creamy Peanut Butter	32g	180	16	3.5	0	0	150	6
Skippy Natural Extra Crunchy Peanut Butter	32g	180	17	0	0	0	125	6
Skippy Super Chunky Peanut Butter	35g	180	12	0	0	0	160	15
Smart Balance Natural Creamy Peanut Butter	32g	200	17	3	0	0	110	5
Smart Balance Natural Chunky Peanut Butter	32g	200	18	3	0	0	110	6
Smucker's Caramel Dessert Topping	41g	120	0	0	0	0	110	29
Smucker's Fruit Jam	20g	50	0	0	0	0	0	13
Smucker's Fruit Jelly	20g	50	0	0	0	0	5	13
Smucker's Fruit Preserves	20g	50	0	0	0	0	0	13
Smucker's Low Sugar Fruit Preserves	17g	25	0	0	0	0	0	6
Smucker's Magic Shell Chocolate Fudge Ice Cream Topping Syrup	34g	210	16	7	0	0	45	17
Smucker's Natural Chunky Peanut Butter	32g	210	16	2.5	0	0	120	6
Smucker's Natural Creamy Peanut Butter	32g	210	16	2.5	0	0	120	6
Smucker's Simply Fruit Spreadable Fruit	19g	40	0	0	0	0	0	10
Smucker's Sugar Free Fruit Jam	17g	10	0	0	0	0	0	5
Smucker's Sugar Free Fruit Preserves	17g	10	0	0	0	0	0	5
Smucker's Sundae Caramel Syrup	40g	100	0	0	0	0	110	25
Soy Vay Oriental Teriyaki Marinade & Sauce	15g	35	1	0	0	0	490	6
Spring Tree Maple Syrup	60ml	210	0	0	0	0	5	53
Sunkist Almond Accents Salad Topping	7g	40	3.5	0	0	0	55	2
Sweet Baby Ray's Barbecue Sauce	37g	70	0	0	0	0	290	18
T. Marzetti Chunky Blue Cheese Salad Dressing	29g	150	15	3	0	15	320	1
T. Marzetti Classic Ranch Salad Dressing	29g	160	17	2.5	0	10	200	1
T. Marzetti Cream Cheese Dip	32g	70	3	2	0	15	85	10
T. Marzetti Dill Dip	29g	120	13	3.5	0	20	200	2
T. Marzetti Original Coleslaw Salad Dressing	32g	160	14	2	0	20	380	6
T. Marzetti Ranch Dip	31g	60	6	1	0	5	240	2

Condiments & Sauces

	Serving	Calories	Total fat (gm)	Saturated fat (gm)	Trans fats (gm)	Cholesterol (mg)	Sodium (mg)	Carbs (gm)
Taco Bell Home Originals Taco Seasoning Mix	6g	20	0	0	0	0	370	3
Tapatio Salsa Picante Hot Sauce	5g	0	0	0	0	0	110	0
Texas Pete Hot Sauce	4g	0	0	0	0	0	100	1
Tostitos Salsa	33g	10	0	0	0	0	250	2
Tostitos Salsa Con Queso Dip	34g	40	2.5	1	0	5	280	5
Tostitos Southwest Ranch Dip	32g	60	5	0.5	0	5	160	2
Tostitos Zesty Bean Dip	33g	45	2	0.5	0	0	230	5
Tribe Classic Hummus	28g	50	3.5	0	0	0	130	4
Vlasic Dill Pickles	28g	5	0	0	0	0	210	1
Vlasic Dill Relish	15g	5	0	0	0	0	240	1
Vlasic Lightly Seasoned Dill Pickle Spears	28g	5	0	0	0	0	210	1
Vlasic Sandwich Stackers Dill Pickles	28g	5	0	0	0	0	210	1
Vlasic Sandwich Stackers Sweet & Spicy Bread & Butter Pickles	28g	30	0	0	0	0	170	7
Vlasic Spicy Dill Pickle Spears	28g	5	0	0	0	0	280	1
Vlasic Super Sandwich Stackers	28g	5	0	0	0	0	210	1
Vlasic Sweet Relish	15g	15	0	0	0	0	140	4
Vlasic Tangy Bread & Butter Pickles	28g	25	0	0	0	0	170	6
Vlasic Tart Dill Pickles	28g	5	0	0	0	0	390	3
Vlasic Gherkin Sweet Pickles	28g	35	0	0	0	0	170	9
Welch's Concord Grape Jam	20g	50	0	0	0	0	10	13
Welch's Concord Grape Jelly	20g	50	0	0	0	0	15	13
Welch's Strawberry Fruit Spread	20g	50	0	0	0	0	10	13
Wholly Guacamole Original Dip	30g	60	5	1	0	0	80	3
Wick Fowlers' 2 Alarm Chili Seasoning Mix	17g	60	1.5	0	0	0	980	10
Wishbone Blue Cheese Salad Dressing	31ml	150	15	2.5	0	5	260	2
Wishbone Deluxe French Salad Dressing	31ml	120	11	1.5	0	0	170	5
Wishbone Italian Salad Dressing	29ml	90	8	1	0	0	490	3
Wishbone Just 2 Good 1/2 Less Fat Italian Salad Dressing	30ml	35	2	0	0	0	350	4
Wishbone Ranch Salad Dressing	30ml	120	13	2	0	5	250	2
Wishbone Robusto Italian Salad Dressing	29ml	90	8	1	0	0	530	3
Wishbone Thousand Island Salad Dressing	31ml	130	12	2	0	10	300	6

Dairy

	Serving	Calories	Total fat (gm)	Saturated fat (gm)	Trans fats (gm)	Cholesterol (mg)	Sodium (mg)	Carbs (gm)
Alouette Cheese Spread	23g	70	6	4	0	15	70	1
Alouette Light Cream Cheese	23g	50	4	2.5	0	15	60	2
Alouette Gournay Cheese Spread	23g	80	8	4.5	0	20	100	1
Alpine Lace Swiss Cheese	23g	70	4.5	3	0	15	90	1
Anderson Erickson 2% Milk	240ml	120	5	3	0	20	120	12
Anderson Erickson Fat Free Milk	245ml	80	0	0	0	5	120	12
Athenos Feta Cheese	28g	80	6	3.5	0	20	330	1
Belgioioso Mozzarella Cheese	28g	80	6	4	0	20	85	0
Belgioioso Parmesan Cheese	5g	20	1	1	0	5	45	0
Belgioioso Plain Cream Cheese	14g	60	6	3.5	0	20	5	0
Benecol Spread	14g	50	5	0.5	0	0	110	0
Benecol Vegetable Oil Spread	14g	70	8	1	0	0	110	0
Blue Bonnet Vegetable Oil Spread	14g	60	7	1	0	0	125	0
Blue Diamond Almond Breeze Original Milk Substitute	240ml	60	2.5	0	0	0	150	8
Borden American Cheese	19g	60	4.5	3	0	15	250	2
Borden Cheddar Cheese	28g	120	10	7	0	30	210	1
Boursin Gournay Cheese Spread	29g	120	12	8	0	30	180	1
Breakstones' 2% Milkfat Cottage Cheese	124g	90	2.5	1.5	0	15	400	6
Breakstones 4% Milkfat Cottage Cheese	124g	120	5	3	0	25	430	6
Breakstones' Fat Free Cottage Cheese	126g	80	0	0	0	10	450	8
Breakstones' Fat Free Sour Cream	32g	30	0	0	0	5	25	5
Breakstones' Live Active 2% Milkfat Cottage Cheese	113g	90	2	1.5	0	15	380	8
Breakstones' Reduced Fat Light Sour Cream	31g	40	3	2	0	15	20	2
Breakstones' Sour Cream	30g	60	5	3.5	0	20	10	1
Breyers Yo-Crunch Low Fat Strawberry Yogurt	170g	200	4.5	2.5	0	10	95	36
Breyers Yo-Crunch Low Fat Vanilla Yogurt	170g	200	4.5	2.5	0	10	95	35
Brummel & Brown Vegetable Oil Spread	14g	45	5	1	0	0	90	0
Cabot Vermont Cheddar Cheese	28g	70	4.5	3	0	15	170	1
Cabot Vermont Pepper Jack Cheese	28g	110	9	6	0	30	170	1
Chobani Nonfat Blueberry Yogurt	170g	140	0	0	0	0	65	20
Chobani Nonfat Peach Yogurt	170g	140	0	0	0	0	80	20
Cool Whip Spray Whipped Topping	6g	15	1	1	0	0	0	2
Crystal Farms Large White Fresh Eggs	1 egg	70	4.5	1.5	0	215	65	1
Daisy 50% Less Fat Light Sour Cream	30g	40	2.5	2	0	10	25	2
Daisy Sour Cream	30g	60	5	3.5	0	20	15	1
Dannon Activia 1.5% Milkfat Flavored Yogurt	113g	110	2	1	0	5	65	19

Dairy

	Serving	Calories	Total fat (gm)	Saturated fat (gm)	Trans fats (gm)	Cholesterol (mg)	Sodium (mg)	Carbs (gm)
Dannon Activia 2% Milkfat Flavored Yogurt	227g	220	4	2.5	0	15	140	37
Dannon Activia Nonfat Light Flavored Yogurt	113g	70	0	0	0	5	65	13
Dannon All Natural Coffee Yogurt	170g	160	2.5	1.5	0	10	105	26
Dannon All Natural Nonfat Plain Yogurt	170g	80	0	0	0	5	115	12
Dannon All Natural Vanilla Yogurt	170g	150	2.5	1.5	0	10	105	25
Dannon Danactive Dairy Drink	94ml	90	1.5	1	0	5	40	16
Dannon Danimals Crush Cups Low Fat Strawberry Yogurt	113g	100	1.5	1	0	10	55	17
Dannon Danimals Yogurt Smoothie	94ml	70	0.5	0	0	5	35	15
Dannon Dan-O-Nino Strawberry Yogurt	50g	60	2	1	0	5	20	7
Dannon Fruit On The Bottom Flavored Yogurt	170g	140	1.5	1	0	5	110	27
Dannon La Creme Yogurt	113g	140	5	3	0	15	65	20
Dannon Light & Fit Blackberry Yogurt	170g	80	0	0	0	5	75	16
Dannon Light & Fit Carb & Sugar Control Strawberries & Cream Yogurt	113g	60	3	2	0	10	25	3
Dannon Light & Fit Nonfat Blueberry Yogurt	170g	80	0	0	0	5	75	16
Dannon Light & Fit Nonfat Peach Yogurt	170g	80	0	0	0	5	75	16
Dannon Light & Fit Nonfat Raspberry Yogurt	170g	80	0	0	0	5	75	16
Dannon Light & Fit Nonfat Strawberry Yogurt	227g	110	0	0	0	5	110	21
Dannon Light & Fit Nonfat Strawberry, Blueberry & Raspberry Yogurt	113g	60	0	0	0	0	55	10
Dannon Light & Fit Nonfat Vanilla Yogurt	170g	80	0	0	0	5	75	16
Dannon Light & Fit Strawberry Banana Yogurt	170g	80	0	0	0	5	75	16
Dannon Light & Fit White Chocolate Raspberry Yogurt	170g	80	0	0	0	5	75	16
Dannon Natural 1.5% Milkfat Vanilla Yogurt	227g	200	3	2	0	15	140	34
Dannon Natural Nonfat Plain Yogurt	227g	150	8	5	0	20	115	12
Dannon Plain Nonfat Yogurt	227g	110	0	0	0	5	150	16
Dannon Premium Low Fat Plain Yogurt	227g	140	3.5	2	0	15	150	16
Dean's 2% Milk	240ml	130	5	3	0	20	130	12
Dean's 4% Milkfat Cottage Cheese	113g	110	5	3	0	25	440	4
Dean's Country Fresh 2% Milk	240ml	130	5	3	0	20	125	12
Dean's Country Fresh Fat Free Milk	1 cup	90	0	0	0	5	125	13
Dean's Country Fresh Whole Milk	240ml	150	8	5	0	35	120	12
Dean's Fat Free Milk	240ml	90	0	0	0	5	130	13
Dean's Low Fat Cottage Cheese	113g	80	1.5	1	0	10	480	4
Dean's Whole Milk	240ml	150	8	5	0	35	120	12
DiGiorno Parmesan Cheese	28g	110	8	4.5	0	25	430	1

Dairy

Dairy	Serving	Calories	Total fat (gm)	Saturated fat (gm)	Trans fats (gm)	Cholesterol (mg)	Sodium (mg)	Carbs (gm)
DiGiorno Parmesan, Romano & Asiago Cheese	28g	110	8	5	0	25	370	1
Earth Balance Vegetable Oil Spread	14g	100	11	3.5	0	0	120	0
Egg Beaters Egg Substitute Real Egg Product	61g	30	0	0	0	0	115	1
Egg Beaters Egg Substitute Whites Only	46g	25	0	0	0	0	75	1
Eggland's Best Large Brown Eggs	50g	70	4	1	0	170	65	0
Eggland's Best Large Brown Organic Eggs	50g	70	4	1	0	170	65	0
Eggs	1 item	63	4	1	0	186	62	0
Fage Total Plain Yogurt	200g	130	4	3	0	10	65	8
Friendship Sour Cream	30g	60	5	3.5	0	20	15	1
Frigo Cheese Heads Mozzarella String Cheese	28g	80	6	3.5	0	15	200	1
Garelick Farms 1% Milk	245ml	110	2.5	1.5	0	10	130	13
Garelick Farms 2% Milk	240ml	130	5	3	0	20	130	12
Garelick Farms Fat Free Milk	240ml	90	0	0	0	5	130	13
Garelick Farms Whole Milk	240ml	150	8	5	0	35	120	12
Hood 1% Milk	236ml	110	2.5	1.5	0	15	125	13
Hood 2% Milk	240ml	130	5	3	0	20	125	13
Hood Fat Free Milk	235ml	80	0	0	0	5	125	13
Hood Lactaid 100 1% Milk	236ml	110	2.5	1.5	0	15	125	13
Hood Lactaid 100 2% Milk	240ml	130	5	3	0	20	125	13
Hood Lactaid 100 Fat Free Milk	240ml	80	0	0	0	5	125	13
Hood Lactaid 100 Whole Milk	244ml	150	8	5	0	35	125	12
Hood Simply Smart 1% Milk	236ml	120	2.5	1.5	0	15	130	13
Hood Simply Smart Fat Free Milk	235ml	90	0	0	0	5	130	13
Hood Whole Milk	236ml	150	8	5	0	35	125	12
Horizon Organic 1% Low Fat Chocolate Milk	240ml	170	3	1.5	0	15	140	27
Horizon Organic 1% Milk	240ml	100	2.5	1.5	0	10	125	12
Horizon Organic 2% Milk	1 cup	120	5	3	0	25	125	12
Horizon Organic Fat Free Milk	240ml	90	0	0	0	5	130	12
Horizon Organic Whole Milk	236ml	150	8	5	0	35	125	12
Hotel Bar Butter	14g	100	11	7	0	30	90	0
I Can't Believe It's Not Butter Light Spread	14g	50	5	0	0	0	85	0
Imperial Margarine	14g	50	5	1	0	0	90	0
Imperial Vegetable Oil Spread	14g	80	8	1.5	2	0	105	0
Kerry Gold Dubliner Cheese Wedge	28g	110	9	6	0	25	210	0
Kraft American Cheese	19g	25	0	0	0	5	250	2
Kraft Cheddar & Mozzarella Cheese	28g	90	7	4.5	0	20	200	1
Kraft Cheddar Cheese	28g	90	6	3.5	0	20	240	1

Dairy

	Serving	Calories	Total fat (gm)	Saturated fat (gm)	Trans fats (gm)	Cholesterol (mg)	Sodium (mg)	Carbs (gm)
Kraft Cheddar Monterey Jack Cheese	28g	100	8	5	0	25	190	1
Kraft Cheddar Processed Cheese	21g	50	3	2	0	10	280	2
Kraft Classic Melts Chedder Monterey Jack & American Cheese	28g	100	8	5	0	30	380	2
Kraft Colby Cheese	28g	110	9	5	0	30	180	1
Kraft Colby Jack Cheese	23g	90	7	4.5	0	25	150	0
Kraft Cracker Barrel Baby Swiss Cheese	28g	110	9	6	0	25	110	0
Kraft Cracker Barrel Cheddar Cheese	28g	110	9	6	0	30	180	1
Kraft Cracker Barrel NY Aged Reserve Cheddar Cheese	28g	120	10	6	0	30	180	0
Kraft Deli Deluxe American Cheese	28g	100	9	5	0	30	460	1
Kraft Deli Deluxe Cheddar Processed Cheese	28g	110	9	5	0	30	450	1
Kraft Easy Cheese American Aerosol Cheese	32g	90	6	2	0	15	420	2
Kraft Easy Cheese Cheddar Aerosol Cheese	32g	80	6	2	0	10	150	2
Kraft Four Cheese Blend Cheese	28g	80	5	3	0	15	240	1
Kraft Free Cheddar Cheese	28g	45	0	0	0	5	280	2
Kraft Free Mozzarella Cheese	28g	45	0	0	0	5	280	2
Kraft Mozzarella & Parmesan Cheese	28g	90	6	4	0	20	210	1
Kraft Mozzarella Cheese	28g	90	6	3.5	0	20	200	1
Kraft Parmesan Cheese	28g	110	8	4.5	0	25	410	1
Kraft Parmesan Romano & Asiago Cheese	28g	110	8	5	0	25	370	1
Kraft Pepper Jack Cheese	28g	110	9	5	0	30	190	1
Kraft Philadelphia Cheesecake Cream Cheese	86g	260	20	12	1	80	300	17
Kraft Philadelphia Flavors Garden Vegetable Cream Cheese	31g	90	8	5	0	35	160	2
Kraft Philadelphia Honey Nut Cream Cheese	32g	90	8	4.5	0	30	110	4
Kraft Philadelphia Onion & Chive Cream Cheese	31g	90	9	5	0	35	150	2
Kraft Philadelphia Original Cream Cheese	28g	100	10	6	0	30	90	1
Kraft Philadelphia Plain Neufchatel Brick	28g	70	6	4	0	20	120	1
Kraft Philadelphia Salmon Cream Cheese	31g	90	8	5	0	30	210	2
Kraft Philadelphia Strawberry Cream Cheese	32g	70	4.5	2.5	0	20	120	6
Kraft Philadelphia Garden Vegetable Cream Cheese	32g	70	5	3.5	0	20	190	2
Kraft Pimento Cream Cheese	32g	80	6	4	0	25	140	3
Kraft Provolone Cheese	28g	100	8	4.5	0	25	230	0
Kraft Shelf Stable Cheddar Cheese	32g	90	8	4.5	0	25	520	1

Dairy	Serving	Calories	Total fat (gm)	Saturated fat (gm)	Trans fats (gm)	Cholesterol (mg)	Sodium (mg)	Carbs (gm)
Kraft Shelf Stable Parmesan & Romano Cheese	5g	20	1.5	1	0	5	85	0
Kraft Shelf Stable Parmesan Cheese	5g	20	1.5	1	0	5	85	0
Kraft Singles American Cheese	19g	60	4.5	2.5	0	15	250	1
Kraft Singles Cheddar Processed Cheese	21g	60	4.5	3	0	15	270	2
Kraft Singles Select American Cheese	19g	70	6	3.5	0	20	310	1
Kraft Snackables Cheddar & Monterey Jack Cheese Cube	30g	90	6	3.5	0	20	270	1
Kraft Snackables Cheddar & Mozzarella Cheese Twist	21g	60	4	2.5	0	15	140	0
Kraft Snackables Cheddar & Mozzarella String Cheese	21g	60	3.5	2	0	10	140	0
Kraft Snackables Colby & Monterey Jack Cheese	30g	110	9	6	0	30	240	1
Kraft Snackables Cracker Cuts Cheddar Cheese	28g	120	10	6	0	30	190	1
Kraft Snackables Cracker Cuts Colby Monterey Jack Cheese	28g	110	9	5	0	30	180	0
Kraft Snackables Mozzarella String Cheese	28g	70	4.5	2.5	0	15	220	1
Kraft Swiss Cheese	23g	90	7	4.5	0	25	40	0
Kraft Taco Cheese	28g	100	8	5	0	25	220	2
Kraft Velveeta American Cheese	28g	80	6	3.5	0	25	400	3
Kraft Velveeta Cheese Loaf	28g	80	6	3.5	0	20	420	3
Kraft Velveeta Shredded Processed Cheese	28g	90	6	4	0	25	330	3
Land O' Lakes American Cheese	21g	70	5	3	0	15	280	2
Land O' Lakes Brown Natural Eggs	1 egg	80	5	1.5	0	240	70	1
Land O' Lakes Butter Blend	14g	50	5	2	0	5	90	0
Land O' Lakes Fresh Buttery Taste Vegetable Oil	14g	70	8	2	0	0	80	0
Land O' Lakes Margarine	14g	100	11	2	2.5	0	105	0
Land O' Lakes Sweet Cream Butter	14g	100	11	7	0	30	95	0
Land O' Lakes Whipped Sweet Cream Butter	7g	50	6	3.5	0	15	50	0
Laughing Cow 50% Less Fat Cheese Spread	21g	35	2	1	0	10	260	1
Laughing Cow Cheddar & Swiss Cheese Spread	21g	35	2	1	0	10	260	1
Laughing Cow Mini Babybel Round Cheddar Cheese	21g	70	6	4	0	20	170	0
Laughing Cow Swiss Cheese Spread	21g	50	4	2.5	0	15	250	1
Lehigh Valley Whole Milk	1 cup	150	8	5	0	35	120	12
Meyenberg Whole White Goat's Milk	240ml	140	7	4	0	25	115	11
Move Over Butter Vegetable Oil Spread	9g	50	6	1	0	0	75	0
Nestle Nesquik 2% Chocolate Milk	250ml	200	5	3.5	0	15	170	30

Dairy

Dairy	Serving	Calories	Total fat (gm)	Saturated fat (gm)	Trans fats (gm)	Cholesterol (mg)	Sodium (mg)	Carbs (gm)
Nestle Nesquik 2% Strawberry Milk	250ml	200	5	3	0	15	120	33
Nestle Nesquik Chocolate Milkshake	240ml	180	5	3	0	20	180	26
Nestle Nesquik Fat Free Chocolate Milk	240ml	150	0	0	0	5	160	29
Odwalla Super Protein Vanilla Almond Soymilk Shake	239ml	190	6	1	0	0	80	25
Organic Valley 1% Milk	236ml	110	2.5	1.5	0	15	130	13
Organic Valley 2% Milk	232ml	130	5	3	0	20	120	12
Organic Valley Fat Free Milk	235ml	90	0	0	0	5	125	13
Organic Valley Large Brown Organic Eggs	50g	60	4	1.5	0	0	70	1
Organic Valley Whole Milk	233ml	150	8	5	0	30	120	12
Papetti Foods All Whites Egg Substitute	56g	30	0	0	0	0	95	1
Parkay Vegetable Oil Spread	14g	80	9	0	0	0	110	0
Polly-O Mozzarella Cheese	28g	70	5	3	0	15	200	1
Prairie Farms 1% Milk	1 cup	100	2.5	1.5	0	15	120	11
Prairie Farms 2% Milk	1 cup	120	5	3.5	0	25	120	11
Prairie Farms Fat Free Milk	1 cup	80	0	0	0	5	120	11
President Brie Cheese	28g	100	9	4	0	20	120	0
President Feta Cheese	28g	35	0	0	0	5	260	1
Promise Activ Supershots Strawberry Yogurt Drink	1 item	70	3.5	0	0	0	25	8
Promise Buttery Spread	14g	80	8	1.5	0	0	85	0
Reddi-Whip Aerosol Whipped Cream	5g	15	1	0.5	0	5	0	1
Reddi-Whip Aerosol Whipped Topping	5g	5	0	0	0	0	0	1
Rice Dream 1% Low Fat Original Rice Drink	240ml	120	2.5	0	0	0	80	23
Rice Dream Original Non Dairy Beverage	243ml	120	2.5	0	0	0	100	23
Rice Dream Vanilla Non Dairy Beverage	243ml	130	2.5	0	0	0	105	26
Roberts' 2% Milk	240ml	120	5	3.5	0	25	120	11
Roberts' Fat Free Milk	240ml	80	0	0	0	5	120	11
Roberts Whole Milk	240ml	150	8	5	0	35	120	11
Rondele Cheese Spread	23g	70	7	5	0	20	135	1
Saladena Goat Cheese	1 cup	80	7	4	0	30	110	0
Sargento Artisan Blends Mozzarella & Provolone Cheese	28g	90	7	4.5	0	20	170	1
Sargento Cheddar Cheese	28g	110	9	5	0	25	190	1
Sargento Colby Jack Cheese	19g	70	6	4	0	15	125	0
Sargento Deli Style Baby Swiss Cheese	19g	70	5	3.5	0	15	40	0
Sargento Deli Style Cheddar Cheese	21g	80	7	4	0	20	140	0
Sargento Deli Style Mozzarella Cheese	21g	60	4	2.5	0	10	140	1
Sargento Deli Style Pepper Jack Cheese	21g	80	6	4	0	20	140	0
Sargento Deli Style Swiss Cheese	19g	70	5	3	0	20	40	0

Dairy

	Serving	Calories	Total fat (gm)	Saturated fat (gm)	Trans fats (gm)	Cholesterol (mg)	Sodium (mg)	Carbs (gm)
Sargento Monterey Jack & Cheddar Cheese	28g	80	6	3	0	20	200	1
Sargento Mozzarella Cheese	28g	80	5	3.5	0	15	190	1
Sargento Mozzarella String Cheese	28g	80	6	3.5	0	15	240	1
Sargento Muenster Cheese	21g	80	6	4	0	20	135	0
Sargento Parmesan Cheese	5g	20	1.5	1	0	5	55	0
Sargento Provolone Cheese	19g	50	3.5	2	0	10	140	0
Sargento Swiss Cheese	21g	60	4	2	0	15	30	1
Schreiber Weight Watchers Mozzarella String Cheese	24g	50	2.5	1	0	5	150	1
Shedd's Country Crock Butter Blend	11g	80	9	3.5	0	15	85	0
Shedd's Country Crock Light Vegetable Oil Spread	14g	50	5	1	0	0	90	0
Shedd's Country Crock Margarine	14g	60	7	1.5	0	0	85	0
Shedd's Country Crock Plus Margarine	14g	50	5	1	0	0	95	0
Shedd's Country Crock Plus Vegetable Oil Spread	14g	50	5	1	0	0	95	0
Shedd's Country Crock Vegetable Oil Spread	14g	60	7	1.5	0	0	110	0
Silk Chocolate Milk Substitute	240ml	140	3	0.5	0	0	100	23
Silk Light Chocolate Milk Substitute	243ml	120	1.5	0	0	0	100	22
Silk Light Plain Milk Substitute	243ml	70	2	0	0	0	120	8
Silk Light Vanilla Milk Substitute	240ml	80	1.5	0	0	0	95	10
Silk Plain Milk Substitute	240ml	100	4	0.5	0	0	120	8
Silk Plus Plain Milk Substitute	240ml	110	5	0.5	0	0	120	8
Silk Plus Vanilla Milk Substitute	243ml	100	3.5	0.5	0	0	95	14
Silk Vanilla Milk Substitute	240ml	100	3.5	0.5	0	0	95	10
Silk Very Vanilla Milk Substitute	240ml	130	4	0.5	0	0	140	19
Smart Balance Light Vegetable Oil Spread	14g	50	5	0	0	0	85	0
Smart Balance Omega Vegetable Oil Spread	13g	80	9	2.5	0	0	85	0
Smart Balance Vegetable Oil Spread	14g	80	9	0	0	0	85	0
Smith's 2% Milk	15ml	120	14	2	0	0	0	0
Sorrento Mozzarella Cheese	30g	90	6	4	0	30	130	0
Sorrento Stringsters Mozzarella String Cheese	28g	70	4	3	0	10	180	1
Stonyfield Farm Chocolate Underground Yogurt	170g	170	0	0	0	0	110	37
Stonyfield Farm Fat Free Milk	244ml	80	0	0	0	5	125	13
Stonyfield Farm French Vanilla Yogurt	170mg	130	0	0	0	0	115	25
Stonyfield Farm Low Fat Plain Yogurt	227g	120	2	1.5	0	10	150	15
Stonyfield Farm Low Fat Vanilla Yogurt	227g	180	2	1	0	10	140	30

Dairy	Serving	Calories	Total fat (gm)	Saturated fat (gm)	Trans fats (gm)	Cholesterol (mg)	Sodium (mg)	Carbs (gm)
Stonyfield Farm Nonfat French Vanilla Yogurt	227g	180	0	0	0	0	150	33
Stonyfield Farm Nonfat Plain Yogurt	227g	110	0	0	0	0	160	16
Stonyfield Farm Plain Yogurt	227g	170	9	6	0	35	135	13
Stonyfield Farm Vanilla Yogurt	170g	130	1.5	1	0	5	105	22
Stonyfield Farm Whole Milk	236ml	150	8	5	0	35	125	12
Stonyfield Farm Yobaby Peach & Pear Yogurt	113g	110	4	0	0	0	65	13
Swiss Valley Farms 2% Milk	244ml	120	5	3	0	20	120	11
The Organic Cow of Vermont 1% Milk	236ml	110	2.5	1.5	0	15	130	13
The Organic Cow of Vermont Fat Free Milk	235ml	90	0	0	0	5	130	13
Toft's 2% Milk	15ml	120	14	2	0	0	0	0
Treasure Cave Blue Cheese	28g	100	8	5	0	25	380	1
Yoplait Fiber One Nonfat Strawberry & Peach Yogurt	113g	80	0	0	0	5	65	19
Yoplait Kids Flavored Low Fat Yogurt	113g	100	2	1.5	0	10	70	17
Yoplait Kids Flavored Yogurt Drink	92ml	70	1.5	1	0	5	40	11
Yoplait Light Apple Turnover Yogurt	170g	100	0	0	0	5	85	19
Yoplait Light Apricot Mango Yogurt	170g	100	0	0	0	5	85	19
Yoplait Light Berries N' Cream Yogurt	170g	100	0	0	0	5	85	19
Yoplait Light Blackberry Yogurt	170g	100	0	0	0	5	85	19
Yoplait Light Blueberry Patch Yogurt	170g	100	0	0	0	5	85	19
Yoplait Light Boston Cream Pie Yogurt	170g	110	0	0	0	5	90	20
Yoplait Light Harvest Peach Yogurt	170g	100	0	0	0	5	85	19
Yoplait Light Key Lime Pie Yogurt	170g	100	0	0	0	5	85	19
Yoplait Light Lemon Cream Pie Yogurt	170g	110	0	0	0	5	90	20
Yoplait Light Nonfat Strawberry Yogurt	170g	100	0	0	0	5	85	19
Yoplait Light Orange Creme Yogurt	170g	100	0	0	0	5	85	19
Yoplait Light Pineaple Upside Down Cake Yogurt	170g	110	0	0	0	5	90	20
Yoplait Light Red Raspberry Yogurt	170g	100	0	0	0	5	85	19
Yoplait Light Strawberries N' Bananas Yogurt	170g	100	0	0	0	5	85	19
Yoplait Light Thick & Creamy French Vanilla Yogurt	170g	100	0	0	0	5	90	20
Yoplait Light Thick & Creamy Key Lime Pie Yogurt	170g	100	0	0	0	5	90	20
Yoplait Light Thick & Creamy Lemon Meringue Yogurt	170g	100	0	0	0	5	90	20
Yoplait Light Thick & Creamy Mixed Berry Yogurt	170g	100	0	0	0	5	90	20
Yoplait Light Thick & Creamy Nonfat Strawberry Yogurt	170g	100	0	0	0	5	90	20

Dairy

	Serving	Calories	Total fat (gm)	Saturated fat (gm)	Trans fats (gm)	Cholesterol (mg)	Sodium (mg)	Carbs (gm)
Yoplait Light Thick & Creamy Peaches N' Cream Yogurt	170g	100	0	0	0	5	90	20
Yoplait Light Very Cherry Yogurt	170g	100	0	0	0	5	85	19
Yoplait Light Very Vanilla Yogurt	170g	110	0	0	0	5	90	20
Yoplait Original Flavored Yogurt	170g	170	1.5	1	0	10	80	33
Yoplait Thick & Creamy Flavored Yogurt	170g	180	2.5	1.5	0	15	110	31
Yoplait Trix Low Fat Flavored Yogurt	113g	90	0.5	0.5	0	5	50	18
Yoplait Whips Low Fat Chocolate Yogurt	113g	160	4	2.5	0	15	105	25
Yoplait Whips Orange Creme Yogurt	113g	140	2.5	2	0	10	75	25
Yoplait Whips Strawberry Mist Yogurt	113g	140	2.5	0	0	10	75	25
Yoplait Yo Plus Low Fat Flavored Yogurt	113g	110	1.5	1	0	10	70	21
Yoplait Go-Gurt Flavored Yogurt	64g	70	0.5	0	0	5	30	13

Grocery Food Factoid:

Foods found in their natural form are full of phytochemicals—health promoting chemicals only found in plants. When whole foods are processed, many of the phytochemicals are removed. When you eat whole foods you get all the nutrition mother nature intended. Most green colored foods in this guide have lots of phytochemicals.

Grocery Food Factoid:

Of the top 100 most salty foods in this guide 86 % are frozen foods and packaged dinners. These foods are highly processed and contain more sodium than any other category. If you eat packaged dinners or frozen dinners, choose those colored green.

SHOPPING LIST/NOTES:

_____
_____
_____
_____
_____
_____
_____
_____
_____
_____
_____
_____

Frozen Foods

	Serving	Calories	Total fat (gm)	Saturated fat (gm)	Trans fats (gm)	Cholesterol (mg)	Sodium (mg)	Carbs (gm)
Alexia Frozen Julienne Sweet Potato Fries	85g	150	6	0.5	0	0	140	24
Amy's Frozen Cheese Enchilada Entrée	127g	240	14	6	0	35	440	18
Amy's Frozen Organic Cheese Pizza	123g	310	12	4	0	15	590	38
Amy's Frozen Organic Pesto Pizza	128g	310	12	3.5	0	10	480	39
Amy's Frozen Organic Spinach Pizza	132g	310	12	4	0	15	590	38
Amy's Frozen Vegetable Lasagna Entrée	269g	310	12	4.5	0	20	680	35
Armour Homestyle Frozen Beef & Pork Meatballs	85g	260	21	8	0.5	30	640	7
Athen's Foods Frozen Plain Fillo Dough	57g	180	1	0	0	0	220	37
Aunt Jemima Frozen Pancake Breakfast Entrée	103g	220	4	1	0	20	460	40
Bagel Bites Frozen Cheese, Pepperoni & Sausage Bagel Snack Bites	88g	210	7	3	0	14	410	30
Bagel Bites Frozen Pepperoni & Cheese Bagel Snack Bites	88g	220	7	3	0	15	480	30
Bagel Bites Frozen Three Cheese Bagel Snack Bites	88g	210	6	3	0	15	400	30
Banquet Brown N' Serve Frozen Beef Breakfast Sausage	54g	190	17	8	1	15	420	1
Banquet Brown N' Serve Frozen Maple Pork & Turkey Breakfast Sausage	60g	210	19	6	0	25	520	2
Banquet Brown N' Serve Frozen Pork & Turkey Breakfast Sausage	50g	170	15	5	0	25	410	2
Banquet Brown N' Serve Frozen Turkey Breakfast Sausage	60g	110	7	2	0	40	390	2
Banquet Frozen Beef, Corn & Potato Chicken Fried Steak Dinner	283g	380	17	5	0	20	1060	42
Banquet Frozen Chicken Dinner	120g	330	21	5	1.5	75	890	12
Banquet Frozen Chicken Fingers & Fries Dinner	201g	490	20	4.5	0	50	730	59
Banquet Frozen Chicken Nuggets	85g	220	13	2.5	0	25	530	15
Banquet Frozen Chicken Tenders	85g	210	11	2	0	15	430	14
Banquet Frozen Chicken, Corn & Fries Dinner	191g	330	15	3.5	0	25	650	33
Banquet Frozen Fish Sticks Dinner	207g	330	12	3	0	20	560	46
Banquet Frozen Macaroni & Cheese Entrée	340g	390	9	4.5	0	20	1180	60
Banquet Frozen Meatloaf, Mashed Potato & Vegetable Dinner	269g	280	13	5	0	40	1000	28
Banquet Frozen Salisbury Steak Entrée	127g	190	14	6	0.5	25	740	9
Banquet Frozen Salisbury Steak, Mashed Potatoes & Corn Dinner	269g	290	16	7	1	30	1100	25
Banquet Frozen Turkey Pot Pie Oven Bake Dinner	198g	370	21	8	0	30	980	35
Banquet Frozen Turkey, Stuffing, Potato & Vegetable Dinner	262g	280	7	1.5	0	20	1150	41

Frozen Foods

	Serving	Calories	Total fat (gm)	Saturated fat (gm)	Trans fats (gm)	Cholesterol (mg)	Sodium (mg)	Carbs (gm)
Banquet Select Recipes Frozen Chicken, Mashed Potato & Corn Dinner	228g	440	26	6	1.5	80	1140	30
Ben & Jerry's Americone Dream Ice Cream	105g	280	15	10	0	60	95	32
Ben & Jerry's Cherry Garcia Ice Cream	104g	240	14	9	0	60	50	26
Ben & Jerry's Cherry Garcia Lighten Up Yogurt	100g	160	3	2	0	15	60	31
Ben & Jerry's Chocolate Chip Cookie Dough Ice Cream	88g	220	12	9	0	50	80	26
Ben & Jerry's Chocolate Fudge Brownie Cup Ice Cream	88g	220	11	7	0	30	65	27
Ben & Jerry's Chocolate Fudge Brownie Ice Cream	102g	250	12	8	0	35	75	31
Ben & Jerry's Chunky Monkey Ice Cream	107g	290	17	10	0	55	45	30
Ben & Jerry's Cinnamon Buns Ice Cream	111g	290	15	9	0	60	120	36
Ben & Jerry's Coffee Heath Bar Crunch Ice Cream	104g	280	17	10	0	60	110	29
Ben & Jerry's Everything But The ... 2 Twisted Ice Cream	109g	300	19	11	0	50	80	31
Ben & Jerry's Half Baked 2 Twisted Ice Cream	103g	270	13	8	0	45	85	33
Ben & Jerry's Half Baked Lighten Up Yogurt	99g	180	3	1.5	0	20	95	35
Ben & Jerry's Imagine Whirled Peach Ice Cream	100g	270	16	11	0	65	105	28
Ben & Jerry's Karamel Sutra Ice Cream	107g	270	14	9	0	50	75	32
Ben & Jerry's Mint Chocolate Cookie Ice Cream	100g	250	14	8	0	60	100	26
Ben & Jerry's New York Super Fudge Chunk Ice Cream	106g	300	19	11	0	35	55	29
Ben & Jerry's One Cheesecake Brownie Ice Cream	103g	250	15	9	0	70	90	26
Ben & Jerry's Peanut Butter Cup Ice Cream	108g	340	23	11	0	55	125	29
Ben & Jerry's Phish Food Ice Cream	102g	270	12	9	0	25	80	39
Ben & Jerry's Pistachio Ice Cream	104g	250	16	9	0	65	55	22
Ben & Jerry's Strawberry Cheesecake Ice Cream	105g	260	15	8	0	55	50	28
Ben & Jerry's Vanilla Heath Bar Crunch Ice Cream	104g	290	17	11	0	65	110	29
Ben & Jerry's Vanilla Ice Cream	103g	230	14	9	0	70	60	21
Bertolli Frozen Chicken & Pasta Entrée	340g	500	25	11	0.5	125	1360	40
Bertolli Frozen Chicken Florentine & Farfalle Entrée	340g	570	31	17	1.5	175	1040	40
Bertolli Frozen Chicken Parmigian & Penne Entrée	340g	490	22	6	1	40	1330	52
Bertolli Frozen Roasted Chicken & Linguine Entrée	340g	410	17	4.5	0	75	1680	41

Frozen Foods

Frozen Foods	Serving	Calories	Total fat (gm)	Saturated fat (gm)	Trans fats (gm)	Cholesterol (mg)	Sodium (mg)	Carbs (gm)
Bertolli Frozen Shrimp Scampi & Linguini Entrée	340g	550	24	11	0.5	130	990	58
Bertolli Frozen Shrimp, Asparagus & Penne Entrée	340g	440	17	8	0.5	90	980	50
Bertolli Mediterranean Style Frozen Chicken, Broccoli & Rigatoni Entrée	340g	380	15	4	0	40	970	37
Bertolli Oven Bake Meals Frozen Chicken Penne Pasta Entrée	340g	500	26	4.5	0	35	1000	44
Bertolli Oven Bake Meals Frozen Meat Lasagna Rustica Entrée	340g	520	31	13	0	60	1100	35
Bertolli Oven Bake Meals Frozen Tri Color Four Cheese Ravioli Entrée	340g	630	33	20	0.5	115	1190	51
Bird's Eye C & W Frozen Green Peas	87g	70	0	0	0	0	200	12
Bird's Eye Farm Fresh Frozen Peppers & Onions	84g	25	0	0	0	0	10	5
Bird's Eye Frozen Broccoli	87g	30	0	0	0	0	20	4
Bird's Eye Frozen Carrots, Peas, Corn, & Green Beans	86g	60	0	0	0	0	60	12
Bird's Eye Frozen Corn	93g	100	1	0	0	0	0	20
Bird's Eye Frozen Spinach	81g	30	0	0	0	0	125	3
Bird's Eye Frozen Sweet Peas	87g	70	0	0	0	0	0	12
Bird's Eye Steamfresh Frozen Asian Medley	93g	50	2	0	0	0	310	6
Bird's Eye Steamfresh Frozen Asparagus, Corn & Carrots	88g	70	0.5	0	0	0	15	13
Bird's Eye Steamfresh Frozen Baby Peas & Mushrooms	116g	80	2	0	0	0	340	12
Bird's Eye Steamfresh Frozen Broccoli & Cauliflower	95g	30	0	0	0	0	25	4
Bird's Eye Steamfresh Frozen Broccoli, Cauliflower & Carrots	84g	30	0	0	0	0	30	5
Bird's Eye Steamfresh Frozen Brown Rice	136g	150	1	0	0	0	5	31
Bird's Eye Steamfresh Frozen Brussels Sprouts	92g	50	0	0	0	0	20	9
Bird's Eye Steamfresh Frozen Chicken, Penne Pasta & Vegetables Entrée	340g	360	10	2.5	0	30	1030	45
Bird's Eye Steamfresh Frozen Chicken, Rigatoni Pasta & Vegetable Entrée	340g	340	13	5	0	60	880	37
Bird's Eye Steamfresh Frozen Corn On The Cob	85g	90	1	0	0	0	0	19
Bird's Eye Steamfresh Frozen Corn, Carrots, Peas & Green Beans	90g	60	0	0	0	0	20	12
Bird's Eye Steamfresh Frozen Shrimp, Penne Pasta & Vegetable Entrée	340g	450	24	14	0	130	770	39
Bird's Eye Steamfresh Frozen Shrimp, Vegetables & Bowtie Pasta Entrée	340g	420	12	7	0	100	900	55
Bird's Eye Steamfresh Frozen Southwest Blend	83g	90	2	0	0	0	260	16

Frozen Foods

	Serving	Calories	Total fat (gm)	Saturated fat (gm)	Trans fats (gm)	Cholesterol (mg)	Sodium (mg)	Carbs (gm)
Bird's Eye Steamfresh Frozen Sweet Peas	92g	70	0	0	0	0	0	13
Bird's Eye Steamfresh Frozen White Long Grain Rice	85g	160	0	0	0	0	0	36
Bird's Eye Steamfresh Frozen White Vegetable & Long Grain Rice Side Dish	175g	190	0.5	0	0	0	15	42
Bird's Eye Steamfresh Frozen Green Beans	81g	30	0	0	0	0	0	5
Bird's Eye Steamfresh Frozen Green Peas	89g	70	0	0	0	0	0	12
Bird's Eye Voila Frozen Chicken, Vegetables & Pasta Entrée	205g	280	12	7	0	55	600	27
Bird's Eye Voila Frozen Chicken, Vegetables & Three Cheese Pasta Entrée	205g	210	8	3	0.5	30	940	21
Bird's Eye Voila Frozen Pasta with Shrimp Scampi & Vegetable Entrée	222g	190	2.5	1	0	60	540	31
Bird's Eye Voila Frozen Garlic Chicken, Vegetable & Pasta Entrée	178g	240	8	2	1	20	540	29
Bob Evans Garlic Potato Side Dish	124g	140	5	2.5	0	10	430	19
Boca Frozen Soy Protein Burger	71g	120	5	1.5	0	5	380	6
Boca Frozen Vegetable Burger	71g	70	0.5	0	0	0	280	6
Boston Market Frozen Beef & Noodle Entrée	396g	470	12	4	0	80	1310	59
Boston Market Frozen Chicken Parmesan & Spaghetti Entrée	453g	620	24	8	0.5	50	1580	69
Boston Market Frozen Chicken Pot Pie	227g	560	36	13	0	55	930	43
Boston Market Frozen Meatloaf & Mashed Potato Entrée	453g	710	42	16	2.5	95	1590	53
Boston Market Frozen Pot Roast Entrée	453g	440	19	6	1	65	1520	40
Boston Market Frozen Turkey Breast, Mashed Potatoes & Vegetable Dinner	425g	360	14	3	0.5	55	1570	35
Breyer's Chocolate Chip Cookie Dough Ice Cream	67g	160	8	5	0	15	50	20
Breyer's Butter Pecan Ice Cream	66g	150	10	4.5	0	20	110	14
Breyer's Carb Smart Vanilla Splenda Ice Cream	66g	90	6	3.5	0	15	45	13
Breyer's Cherry Vanilla Ice Cream	66g	130	6	4	0	15	55	18
Breyer's Chocolate Chip Ice Cream	66g	150	8	5	0	20	40	17
Breyer's Chocolate Crackle Ice Cream	66g	160	10	7	0	15	30	15
Breyer's Chocolate Ice Cream	66g	140	7	4.5	0	20	45	17
Breyer's Coffee Ice Cream	62g	130	7	4	0	20	45	15
Breyer's Cookies & Cream Ice Cream	66g	150	7	4.5	0	15	90	19
Breyer's Double Churn Butter Pecan Reduced Fat Ice Cream	61g	110	6	2.5	0	10	105	14
Breyer's Double Churn Creamy Vanilla & Strawberry Light Ice Cream	60g	100	3	2	0	10	50	17
Breyer's Double Churn Creamy Vanilla Fat Free Ice Cream	66g	90	0	0	0	0	50	21

Frozen Foods

	Serving	Calories	Total fat (gm)	Saturated fat (gm)	Trans fats (gm)	Cholesterol (mg)	Sodium (mg)	Carbs (gm)
Breyer's Double Churn Neapolitan Reduced Fat Ice Cream	60g	80	4	2.5	0	10	45	14
Breyer's Double Churn Vanilla Bean Light Ice Cream	66g	110	3.5	2	0	10	50	16
Breyer's Double Churn Vanilla Light Splenda Ice Cream	60g	80	4	2.5	0	10	45	14
Breyer's French Vanilla Ice Cream	66g	140	7	4.5	0	45	35	14
Breyer's Heath English Toffee Ice Cream	72g	160	6	3.5	0	10	130	25
Breyer's Homemade Vanilla Ice Cream	66g	140	7	4.5	0	35	55	16
Breyer's Mint Chocolate Chip Ice Cream	66g	150	8	5	0	15	40	17
Breyer's Mrs. Fields Vanilla Ice Cream Sandwich	55g	190	8	4.5	0	10	125	29
Breyer's Natural Vanilla Ice Cream	66g	130	7	4	0	20	35	14
Breyer's Natural Vanilla Lactose Free Ice Cream	65g	130	7	4.5	0	20	35	14
Breyer's Oreo Cookies & Cream Ice Cream	69g	160	8	4.5	0	20	85	20
Breyer's Peach Ice Cream	66g	120	4.5	3	0	15	30	17
Breyer's Reese's Peanut Butter Cup Ice Cream	73g	160	6	2.5	0	10	110	25
Breyer's Rocky Road Ice Cream	67g	150	8	4.5	0	15	45	20
Breyer's Strawberry Cheesecake Ice Cream	67g	150	6	2.5	0	10	75	22
Breyer's Strawberry Ice Cream	66g	120	5	3	0	15	35	15
Breyer's Swirl Chunk Ice Cream	67g	170	8	4.5	0	20	80	20
Breyer's Take Two Vanilla & Chocolate Ice Cream	66g	130	7	4.5	0	20	40	16
Breyer's Triple Chocolate Ice Cream	66g	140	7	4.5	0	20	65	17
Breyer's Vanilla Fudge Twirl Ice Cream	66g	130	6	3.5	0	15	50	17
Breyer's Vanilla Ice Cream	62g	130	7	4	0	20	50	16
Breyer's Vanilla, Chocolate & Strawberry Ice Cream	66g	130	6	4	0	20	35	15
Breyer's Waffle Cone Ice Cream	61g	130	3	2	0	5	95	22
Bridgford Frozen White Parkerhouse Rolls	57g	160	3	1.5	0	0	280	29
Bubba Burger Frozen Beef Burgers	151g	430	35	15	1.5	115	90	1
California Pizza Kitchen Frozen Crispy Thin For Three Pizza	128g	350	17	8	1	35	730	33
California Pizza Kitchen Frozen Crispy Thin Four Cheese Pizza	127g	340	15	8	1	35	610	33
California Pizza Kitchen Frozen Crispy Thin Margherita Pizza	172g	420	18	8	1.5	30	680	45
California Pizza Kitchen Frozen Rising Crust For Three Pizza	119g	320	15	8	0.5	40	700	29
California Pizza Kitchen Frozen Thin & Crispy Crust For Three Pizza	120g	310	13	5	0.5	35	850	31
Celeste Pizza For One Frozen Crust Single Serving Cheese Pizza	158g	350	17	4	5	0	1090	39

Frozen Foods

	Serving	Calories	Total fat (gm)	Saturated fat (gm)	Trans fats (gm)	Cholesterol (mg)	Sodium (mg)	Carbs (gm)
Chungs Frozen White Meat Chicken Egg Rolls	88g	150	4	1	0	10	420	23
Cole's Frozen Mozzarella Garlic Breadsticks	80g	250	8	4	0	25	350	28
Cole's Frozen Zesty Italian Garlic Bread	50g	170	7	2.5	0	0	280	21
Cole's Frozen Garlic Bread	50g	170	8	2.5	0	5	280	21
Contessa Frozen Chicken Stir-Fry Entrée	227g	180	1.5	0	0	30	590	26
Contessa Frozen Sesame Chicken, Vegetable & Rice Entrée	189g	190	3	1	0	25	135	29
Contessa Frozen Shrimp Primavera Entrée	171g	160	2	0	0	75	240	24
Cool Whip Fat Free Frozen Whipped Topping	9g	15	0	0	0	0	5	3
Cool Whip Frozen Strawberry Whipped Topping	9g	25	1.5	1.5	0	0	0	2
Cool Whip Frozen Whipped Topping	9g	25	1.5	1.5	0	0	2	2
Cool Whip Lite 50% Less Fat Frozen Whipped Topping	9g	20	1	1	0	0	0	3
Cool Whip Sugar Free Frozen Whipped Topping	9g	20	1	1	0	0	0	3
Croissant Pockets Frozen Pepperoni Pizza	127g	370	21	9	0	20	750	33
Delizza Frozen Belgian Chocolate Eclair	84g	280	18	11	0	80	90	26
Delizza Frozen Belgian Pastry	75g	270	22	14	0	115	55	13
DiGiorno Frozen Cheese Stuffed Pepperoni Pizza	150g	380	16	8	0.5	40	1040	40
DiGiorno Frozen Cheese Stuffed Three Meat Pizza	136g	350	16	7	0.5	40	950	34
DiGiorno Frozen Four Cheese Garlic Bread	144g	350	14	5	1	20	580	41
DiGiorno Frozen Pepperoni Garlic Bread	145g	380	17	6	1	25	690	40
DiGiorno Frozen Rising Crust Pepperoni Pizza	134g	330	13	5	0	30	940	40
DiGiorno Frozen Rising Crust Sausage Pepperoni Pizza	143g	350	15	6	0	30	990	40
DiGiorno Frozen Rising Crust Spinach Mushroom Garlic Pizza	143g	300	9	4	0	20	780	40
DiGiorno Frozen Rising Crust Supreme Pizza	155g	360	15	6	0	30	990	41
DiGiorno Frozen Rising Crust Three Meat Pizza	144g	360	15	6	0	30	1000	39
DiGiorno Frozen Thin & Crispy Pepperoni Pizza	125g	320	15	7	0.5	35	790	31
DiGiorno Frozen Thin & Crispy Single Serving Pepperoni Pizza	238g	590	25	11	1	50	1180	64
DiGiorno Frozen Thin & Crispy Supreme Pizza	141g	320	15	6	0.5	30	720	33
DiGiorno Frozen Thin & Crisp Crust Four Meat Pizza	133g	320	14	6	0.5	35	850	32

Frozen Foods

Frozen Foods	Serving	Calories	Total fat (gm)	Saturated fat (gm)	Trans fats (gm)	Cholesterol (mg)	Sodium (mg)	Carbs (gm)
DiGiorno Frozen Traditional Crust Single Serving Four Cheese Pizza	260g	720	30	12	3	35	1190	84
DiGiorno Frozen Traditional Crust Single Serving Pepperoni Pizza	263g	770	35	13	3	50	1410	83
DiGiorno Frozen Garlic Bread Supreme	121g	300	14	5	0.5	20	540	31
DiGiorno Ultimate Frozen Crust Supreme Pizza	150g	350	17	7	0	35	950	35
DiGiorno Ultimate Frozen Thin Crust Four Cheese Pizza	130g	320	14	7	0.5	35	870	34
DiGiorno Ultimate Frozen Thin Crust Four Meat Pizza	142g	380	20	8	0.5	50	1130	34
Dole Frozen Whole Blueberries	140g	70	1	0	0	0	0	17
Dove Bar Frozen Dark Chocolate & Vanilla Ice Cream Bars	78g	260	17	11	0	30	35	26
Dove Bar Frozen Milk Chocolate & Vanilla Ice Cream Bars	78g	260	17	11	0	30	50	25
Dreyer's/Edy's Coconut Frozen Fruit Juice Bars	88g	120	3	2.5	0	0	40	21
Dreyer's/Edy's Dibs Vanilla Bite Frozen Ice Cream	103g	390	29	18	0	25	90	30
Dreyer's/Edy's Frozen Fruit Juice Bars	50g	30	0	0	0	0	0	8
Dreyer's/Edy's Fun Flavors Butter Pecan	65g	130	6	2.5	0	15	120	18
Dreyer's/Edy's Fun Flavors Cookie Dough	65g	150	6	4	0	15	75	23
Dreyer's/Edy's Fun Flavors Spumoni	65g	120	4.5	2.5	0	15	65	19
Dreyer's/Edy's Loaded Chocolate Chip Cookie Dough Ice Cream	54g	130	4.5	2.5	0	10	45	21
Dreyer's/Edy's Loaded Chocolate Chip Mint Brownie Ice Cream	51g	120	4.5	2	0	10	35	18
Dreyer's/Edy's Loaded Chocolate Peanut Butter Cup Ice Cream	54g	140	6	3	0	10	70	18
Dreyer's/Edy's Loaded Cookies & Cream Ice Cream	50g	110	3.5	1.5	0	5	60	18
Dreyer's/Edy's Loaded Nestle Butterfinger Ice Cream	53g	130	5	2	0	5	65	19
Dreyer's/Edy's Slow Churned American Idol Limited Edition Ice Cream	62g	120	4	2	0	20	65	19
Dreyer's/Edy's Slow Churned Fat Free Caramel Praline Crunch Yogurt	63g	120	3.5	2	0	10	45	20
Dreyer's/Edy's Slow Churned Light Butter Pecan Ice Cream	60g	120	5	2	0	20	80	16
Dreyer's/Edy's Slow Churned Light Caramel Delight Ice Cream	62g	120	3.5	2	0	20	50	19
Dreyer's/Edy's Slow Churned Light Chocolate Chip Ice Cream	62g	120	4.5	3	0	20	50	17
Dreyer's/Edy's Slow Churned Light Chocolate Fudge Chunk Ice Cream	62g	120	4.5	3	0	20	50	18

Frozen Foods

	Serving	Calories	Total fat (gm)	Saturated fat (gm)	Trans fats (gm)	Cholesterol (mg)	Sodium (mg)	Carbs (gm)
Dreyer's/Edy's Slow Churned Light Chocolate Ice Cream	60g	110	3.5	2	0	20	45	16
Dreyer's/Edy's Slow Churned Light Coffee Ice Cream	60g	105	3.5	2	0	20	45	15
Dreyer's/Edy's Slow Churned Light Cookie Dough Ice Cream	65g	130	4.5	3	0	20	60	20
Dreyer's/Edy's Slow Churned Light Cookies & Cream Ice Cream	65g	160	8	4.5	0	25	60	19
Dreyer's/Edy's Slow Churned Light Double Fudge Brownie Ice Cream	62g	120	4	2	0	20	50	18
Dreyer's/Edy's Slow Churned Light French Silk Ice Cream	63g	130	4.5	3	0	20	65	19
Dreyer's/Edy's Slow Churned Light French Vanilla Ice Cream	60g	100	3.5	2	0	30	45	15
Dreyer's/Edy's Slow Churned Light Ice Cream Fudge Tracks Ice Cream	62g	120	4.5	3	0	20	45	18
Dreyer's/Edy's Slow Churned Light Mint Chocolate Chip Ice Cream	60g	120	4.5	3	0	20	50	17
Dreyer's/Edy's Slow Churned Light No Sugar Added Splenda Butter Pecan Ice Cream	62g	120	5	2	0	10	80	15
Dreyer's/Edy's Slow Churned Light No Sugar Added Splenda Fudge Tracks Ice Cream	62g	110	4	2.5	0	10	75	16
Dreyer's/Edy's Slow Churned Light No Sugar Added Splenda Triple Chocolate Ice Cream	62g	110	3.5	2	0	10	65	17
Dreyer's/Edy's Slow Churned Light No Sugar Added Splenda Vanilla Ice Cream	62g	90	3	2	0	10	70	13
Dreyer's/Edy's Slow Churned Light Rocky Road Ice Cream	60g	120	4	2	0	20	40	17
Dreyer's/Edy's Slow Churned Light Take The Cake Ice Cream	62g	120	4	2.5	0	20	45	18
Dreyer's/Edy's Slow Churned Light Vanilla Bean Ice Cream	60g	100	3.5	2	0	20	45	15
Dreyer's/Edy's Slow Churned Light Vanilla Ice Cream	60g	100	3.5	2	0	20	45	15
Dreyer's/Edy's Slow Churned Vanilla Yogurt	59g	100	3	1.5	0	10	35	17
Dreyer's/Edy's Strawberry Frozen Fruit Juice Bars	86g	80	0	0	0	0	0	21
Dreyer's/Edy's Strawberry, Raspberry & Tangerine Frozen Fruit Juice Bars	51g	30	0	0	0	0	0	8
Dreyer's/Edy's Grand Chocolate Chip Ice Cream	65g	170	9	6	0	25	45	18
Dreyer's/Edy's Grand Chocolate Ice Cream	65g	150	8	4.5	0	25	35	17
Dreyer's/Edy's Grand Cookies & Cream Ice Cream	65g	160	8	4.5	0	25	60	19

Frozen Foods

	Serving	Calories	Total fat (gm)	Saturated fat (gm)	Trans fats (gm)	Cholesterol (mg)	Sodium (mg)	Carbs (gm)
Dreyer's/Edy's Grand Double Vanilla Ice Cream	70g	140	7	4.5	0	35	40	16
Dreyer's/Edy's Grand French Vanilla Ice Cream	65g	150	9	5	0	50	35	16
Dreyer's/Edy's Grand Mint Chocolate Chip Ice Cream	65g	170	9	6	0	25	45	18
Dreyer's/Edy's Grand Neapolitan Ice Cream	65g	140	7	4.5	0	25	35	16
Dreyer's/Edy's Grand Real Strawberry Ice Cream	65g	130	6	3.5	0	20	30	16
Dreyer's/Edy's Grand Rocky Road Ice Cream	65g	170	10	5	0	25	35	18
Dreyer's/Edy's Grand Vanilla Bean Ice Cream	65g	140	8	5	0	25	35	15
Dreyer's/Edy's Grand Vanilla Ice Cream	65g	140	8	4.5	0	25	35	15
Edward's Frozen Chocolate Cream Pie	120g	450	27	17	0	10	330	48
Edward's Frozen Key Lime Pie	92g	330	16	10	2	35	240	43
Edward's Frozen Lemon Meringue Pie	124g	350	8	3.5	0.5	60	250	62
Edward's Frozen Oreo Cream Pie	123g	480	30	17	3.5	10	320	50
Edward's Frozen Turtle Pie	108g	390	22	11	2.5	10	270	46
Edward's Frozen Georgia Pecan Pie	113g	490	26	4.5	3.5	75	280	60
El Monterey Frozen Beef & Bean Green Chili Burrito	113g	290	14	5	0	15	300	32
El Monterey Frozen Beef & Bean Burrito	113g	300	14	5	0	15	300	33
El Monterey Frozen Shredded Beef with Cheese Taquito	128g	350	17	2.5	0	15	540	36
El Monterey Frozen Grilled Chicken & Cheese Taquito	128g	350	18	2.5	0	15	580	36
Eskimo Pie Frozen Vanilla Ice Cream Bar	51g	160	11	8	0	15	35	14
Fast Fixin' Frozen Chicken Bites	89g	210	12	2	0	15	610	16
Fast Fixin' Frozen Chicken Nuggets	85g	190	10	0	0	20	580	16
Fast Fixin' Frozen Chicken Patties	85g	190	10	0	0	20	580	16
Fast Fixin' Frozen Chicken Strips	85g	190	10	0	0	20	580	16
Fast Fixin' Frozen Popcorn Chicken	85g	190	8	1	0	15	660	15
Foster Farms Frozen Chicken Frank Corndogs	75g	180	9	2.5	0	25	540	19
Freschetta Frozen Bake & Rise Four Cheese Pizza	140g	360	13	7	0	25	850	43
Freschetta Frozen Bake & Rise Supreme Pizza	132g	320	13	5	0	25	890	37
Freschetta Frozen Fire Baked Crust Five Cheese Pizza	131g	340	15	6	0	25	780	37
Freschetta Frozen Fire Baked Crust Pepperoni Pizza	154g	410	20	8	0.5	40	1120	38
Freschetta Frozen Fire Baked Crust Supreme Pizza	151g	360	16	6	0	30	840	39

Frozen Foods

	Serving	Calories	Total fat (gm)	Saturated fat (gm)	Trans fats (gm)	Cholesterol (mg)	Sodium (mg)	Carbs (gm)
Freschetta Pizzamore Frozen Crust Large Pepperoni Duo Pizza	89g	240	11	4.5	0	20	620	25
Freschetta Pizzamore Frozen Crust Large Pizza	96g	240	10	4.5	0	20	600	25
Fudgesicle Frozen Fudge Bars	43g	60	1.5	1	0	0	50	12
Fudgesicle Triple Chocolate Frozen Fudge Bars	43g	60	1.5	1	0	0	50	12
Good Humor Strawberry Shortcake Ice Cream Bars	59g	170	9	4	0	5	40	21
Gorton's Frozen Battered Pollock	108g	260	17	3	0	30	770	17
Gorton's Frozen Beer Battered Pollock	103g	230	14	3.5	0	25	550	20
Gorton's Frozen Breaded Pollock	108g	240	12	3	0	30	500	23
Gorton's Frozen Breaded Tilapia	113g	250	12	3.5	0	25	480	23
Gorton's Frozen Potato Breaded Whitefish	103g	240	14	4	0	25	790	20
Gorton's Frozen Whole Shrimp Temptations	113g	120	5	1	0	70	500	8
Gorton's Grilled Pollack Fillets	108g	100	3	0.5	0	70	290	1
Great Range Frozen Ground Buffalo	113g	190	11	4	0	60	60	0
Green Giant Frozen Broccoli	110g	60	2.5	1	0	0	460	7
Green Giant Frozen Broccoli & Rice Side Dish	283g	270	4.5	1.5	0	5	970	52
Green Giant Frozen Broccoli, Cauliflower & Carrots	101g	45	1	0	0	0	380	7
Green Giant Frozen Brussels Sprouts	104g	60	1	0.5	0	5	320	9
Green Giant Frozen Butter Corn	123g	110	2	1	0	5	370	21
Green Giant Frozen Cauliflower	98g	50	2.5	1	0	0	410	6
Green Giant Frozen Cheese Broccoli	110g	45	1.5	0.5	0	0	420	7
Green Giant Frozen Corn	112g	110	2	1	0	5	340	22
Green Giant Frozen Corn On The Cob	½ ear	70	0.5	0	0	0	5	14
Green Giant Frozen Creamed Spinach	109g	70	2.5	1.5	0	0	510	9
Green Giant Frozen Spinach	100g	25	0	0	0	0	200	3
Green Giant Frozen Garden Medley	120g	70	0.5	0	0	0	220	14
Green Giant Healthy Vision Frozen Carrots, Zucchini & Green Beans	109g	45	2	1	0	5	220	6
Green Giant Healthy Weight Frozen Vegetables	110g	90	2.5	1	0	5	240	14
Green Giant Immunity Blend Frozen Broccoli, Carrots, Red & Yellow Peppers	110g	50	3	0	0	0	115	7
Green Giant Just For One Frozen Broccoli	120g	60	3	1	0	0	470	7
Green Giant Nibblers Frozen Corn On The Cob	½ ear	70	0.5	0	0	0	5	14
Green Giant Simply Steam Frozen Carrots, Cauliflower & Sugar Snap Peas	103g	40	1	0	0	5	250	9
Green Giant Simply Steam Frozen Sweet Peas	90g	60	0.5	0	0	0	190	13

Frozen Foods

	Serving	Calories	Total fat (gm)	Saturated fat (gm)	Trans fats (gm)	Cholesterol (mg)	Sodium (mg)	Carbs (gm)
Green Giant Simply Steam Frozen Garden Medley	99g	50	0.5	0	0	0	280	11
Green Giant Simply Steam Frozen Green Beans	81g	45	2	0	0	0	95	5
Green Giant Valley Fresh Steamers Frozen Butter Roasted Red Potatoes	139g	80	1	0.5	0	0	330	16
Green Giant Valley Fresh Steamers Frozen Cheese Broccoli	106g	45	1.5	0	0	0	380	7
Green Giant Valley Fresh Steamers Frozen Corn	83g	90	1	0	0	0	0	19
Haagen-Dazs Butter Pecan Ice Cream	106g	310	23	11	0.5	110	110	21
Haagen-Dazs Caramel Ice Cream Cones	111g	320	19	10	0.5	100	190	32
Haagen-Dazs Chocolate Chocolate Chip Ice Cream	106g	300	20	12	0.5	105	55	26
Haagen-Dazs Chocolate Ice Cream Cup	102g	260	17	10	0.5	100	45	22
Haagen-Dazs Chocolate Ice Cream	106g	270	18	11	0.5	115	60	22
Haagen-Dazs Chocolate Peanut Butter Ice Cream	109g	360	24	11	0	100	100	27
Haagen-Dazs Coffee Ice Cream	106g	270	18	11	0.5	120	70	21
Haagen-Dazs Dulce De Leche Ice Cream	103g	270	16	10	0.5	90	75	27
Haagen-Dazs Fat Free Sorbet	114g	150	0	0	0	0	10	37
Haagen-Dazs Low Fat Vanilla Yogurt	106g	180	2.5	1	0	50	50	31
Haagen-Dazs Pineapple Coconut Ice Cream	95g	230	13	8	0.5	90	55	25
Haagen-Dazs Rum Raisin Ice Cream	106g	260	17	10	0.5	100	45	22
Haagen-Dazs Strawberry Ice Cream	104g	250	16	9	0.5	85	45	23
Haagen-Dazs Vanilla Bean Ice Cream	106g	290	18	11	0.5	105	75	26
Haagen-Dazs Vanilla Ice Cream	106g	270	18	11	0.5	120	70	21
Haagen-Dazs Vanilla Ice Cream Bars	87g	310	22	13	0	65	40	22
Haagen-Dazs Vanilla Ice Cream Cups	104g	260	17	10	0.5	105	50	21
Haagen-Dazs Vanilla Swiss Almond Ice Cream	103g	300	20	10	0.5	95	60	24
Healthy Choice Cafe Steamers Frozen Beef, Potato & Vegetable Entrée	284g	230	8	2	0	35	600	21
Healthy Choice Cafe Steamers Frozen Beef, Vegetable & Rice Entrée	289g	310	5	1.5	0	30	600	49
Healthy Choice Cafe Steamers Frozen Chicken, Shrimp, Rice & Vegetable Entrée	295g	260	4	1	0	50	570	40
Healthy Choice Cafe Steamers Frozen Chicken, Vegetable & Pasta Cheese Entrée	284g	320	7	1.5	0	35	580	45
Healthy Choice Cafe Steamers Frozen Chicken, Vegetable & Pasta Entrée	301g	320	9	2.5	0	35	580	39
Healthy Choice Cafe Steamers Frozen Chicken, Vegetable & Rice Entrée	286g	290	4	1	0	30	480	46
Healthy Choice Cafe Steamers Frozen Steak, Potato & Vegetable Entrée	269g	260	4	1.5	0	35	580	36

Frozen Foods

	Serving	Calories	Total fat (gm)	Saturated fat (gm)	Trans fats (gm)	Cholesterol (mg)	Sodium (mg)	Carbs (gm)
Healthy Choice Cafe Steamers Frozen Grilled Chicken, Vegetable & Pasta Entrée	284g	270	4.5	1.5	0	30	550	35
Healthy Choice Complete Selections Frozen Beef, Mashed Potatoes & Vegetable Entrée	319g	260	6	2	0	45	600	33
Healthy Choice Complete Selections Frozen Chicken, Mashed Potatoes & Vegetable Entrée	301g	360	9	1.5	0	25	530	53
Healthy Choice Complete Selections Frozen Chicken, Vegetable & Fettuccini Entrée	329g	370	9	2	0	25	590	54
Healthy Choice Complete Selections Frozen Chicken, Vegetable & Rice Entrée	340g	390	10	1.5	0	20	500	61
Healthy Choice Complete Selections Frozen Fish Pilaf & Dessert Entrée	303g	320	6	1.5	0	25	460	51
Healthy Choice Complete Selections Frozen Meatloaf, Potato, Vegetable & Dessert Entrée	340g	300	7	2.5	0	35	530	44
Healthy Choice Complete Selections Frozen Salisbury Steak, Potato, Vegetable & Dessert Entrée	354g	290	6	2	0	35	520	42
Healthy Choice Complete Selections Frozen Turkey & Vegetable & Dessert Entrée	298g	280	4	1	0	30	450	41
Healthy Choice Complete Selections Frozen Turkey, Sweet Potato & Vegetable Entrée	306g	320	3.5	1.5	0	35	530	53
Healthy Choice Frozen Fudge Bars	64g	80	1.5	1	0	5	65	13
Healthy Choice Simple Selections Frozen Chicken, Vegetable & Rice Entrée	241g	310	4.5	1	0	25	310	53
Healthy Choice Simple Selections Frozen Turkey, Mashed Potato & Vegetable Entrée	241g	220	5	1.5	0	35	500	28
Home Market Cooked Perfect Frozen Beef Meatballs	85g	240	19	7	0.5	60	460	5
Hot Pockets Frozen 4 Meat 4 Cheese Pizza Pockets	127g	340	16	7	0	30	650	37
Hot Pockets Frozen 4 Meat & 4 Cheese Calzones	120g	290	12	5	0	25	830	33
Hot Pockets Frozen Barbeque Sauce with Beef Pockets	127g	310	10	4.5	0	25	780	43
Hot Pockets Frozen Beef & Cheddar Pockets	127g	320	15	7	0	30	630	36
Hot Pockets Frozen Beef Taco Pockets	127g	290	12	6	0	25	680	34
Hot Pockets Frozen Bruschetta Chicken Paninis	106g	190	6	2.5	0	30	600	25
Hot Pockets Frozen Chicken Melt Pockets	127g	300	12	5	0	30	570	36
Hot Pockets Frozen Egg & Pastry Breakfast Sandwiches	127g	330	15	8	0	70	510	35
Hot Pockets Frozen Egg, Ham & Cheese Breakfast Sandwiches	127g	310	15	7	0	55	350	35

Frozen Foods

	Serving	Calories	Total fat (gm)	Saturated fat (gm)	Trans fats (gm)	Cholesterol (mg)	Sodium (mg)	Carbs (gm)
Hot Pockets Frozen Four Cheese Pizza Pockets	127g	320	13	7	0	25	760	37
Hot Pockets Frozen Ham & Cheese Pockets	127g	260	9	2.5	0	30	820	34
Hot Pockets Frozen Ham & Swiss Paninis	106g	220	8	3.5	0	20	650	26
Hot Pockets Frozen Meatball Mozzarella Pockets	127g	340	16	7	0	30	570	36
Hot Pockets Frozen Pepperoni & 3 Cheese Calzones	120g	310	15	6	0	25	850	33
Hot Pockets Frozen Pepperoni Pizza Pockets	127g	360	19	7	0	35	830	34
Hot Pockets Frozen Philly Steak & Cheese Pockets	127g	310	13	6	0	30	590	37
Hot Pockets Frozen Sausage, Egg & Cheese Breakfast Sandwiches	63g	160	8	4	0	30	200	17
Hot Pockets Frozen Steak & Cheddar Paninis	106g	220	8	4.5	0	25	500	25
Hot Pockets Frozen Supreme Calzones	120g	280	12	4.5	0	20	770	33
Hungry Man Frozen Bourbon Beef Steak, Rice & Green Beans Dinner	454g	620	14	2	0	55	2210	95
Jack's Original Frozen Crust For Three Cheese Pizza	142g	320	13	6	0	30	610	38
Jack's Original Frozen Crust For Three Pizza	156g	390	19	8	0	45	890	38
Jack's Original Frozen Crust Sausage & Pepperoni Pizza	122g	300	15	6	0	35	660	29
Jack's Original Frozen Crust Supreme Pizza	128g	300	15	6	0	35	650	29
Jeno's Crisp N' Tasty Frozen Crisp Crust Single Serving Cheese Pizza	195g	450	21	3.5	6	0	1020	51
Jeno's Crisp N' Tasty Frozen Crisp Crust Single Serving Pepperoni Pizza	192g	490	25	6	4.5	15	1180	50
Jeno's Crisp N' Tasty Frozen Crispy Crust Single Serving Combination Pizza	198g	480	25	6	4.5	15	1140	50
Jimmy Dean Breakfast Bowls Frozen Egg , Potato & Sausage Breakfast	227g	490	34	14	1.5	375	1210	20
Jimmy Dean Breakfast Bowls Frozen Egg, Bacon, Potato & Cheese Breakfast	227g	520	33	13	1.5	395	1490	21
Jimmy Dean Breakfast Bowls Frozen Egg, Potato, Ham & Cheese Breakfast	227g	390	23	9	0	360	1200	23
Jimmy Dean Frozen Biscuit Breakfast Sandwich	102g	320	18	7	3	100	800	27
Jimmy Dean Frozen Croissant Breakfast Sandwich	128g	420	28	9	3	125	820	30
Jimmy Dean Frozen Pancake & Sausage Breakfast Entrée	71g	220	13	4	0	20	350	21
Jimmy Dean Frozen Pork Sausage	56g	180	16	5	0	40	450	1
Jimmy Dean Skillets Frozen Sausage & Potato Breakfast Entrée	127g	220	15	5	0	25	590	16

Frozen Foods

	Serving	Calories	Total fat (gm)	Saturated fat (gm)	Trans fats (gm)	Cholesterol (mg)	Sodium (mg)	Carbs (gm)
Jimmy Dean D-Lights Frozen Muffin Breakfast Sandwich	145g	260	7	3.5	0	35	840	30
Jose Ole Frozen Beef & Cheese Taco	85g	210	11	4	0	20	440	19
Jose Ole Frozen Chicken & Cheese Taquito	85g	230	10	2	0	15	510	27
Jose Ole Frozen Chicken Chimichanga	142g	330	12	3	0	20	550	44
Jose Ole Frozen Chicken Taquito	85g	200	8	1.5	0	10	390	26
Jose Ole Frozen Shredded Steak Taquito	85g	210	9	2	0	10	420	25
Jose Ole Frozen Steak & Cheese Taquito	85g	240	12	3	0	15	470	28
Kashi Frozen Thin Crust Mushroom Trio & Spinach Pizza	113g	250	9	4.5	0	25	660	28
Kashi Frozen Thin Crust Roasted Vegetable Pizza	116g	250	9	4	0	20	630	28
Kashi Frozen Thin Crust Tomato, Garlic & Cheese Pizza	113g	260	9	4	0	20	630	29
Kashi Go Lean Frozen Blueberry Waffles	84g	170	3	0	0	0	300	33
Kashi Go Lean Frozen Original Waffles	84g	170	3	0	0	0	330	33
Keebler Cake Ice Cream Cup	5g	15	0	0	0	0	20	4
Keebler Sugar Ice Cream Cone	13g	50	0.5	0	0	0	55	10
Kellogg's Eggo Bakeshop Swirlz Frozen Toaster Pastries	63g	140	3	1	0	10	270	27
Kellogg's Eggo French Toaster Sticks	90g	220	6	1.5	0	25	540	35
Kellogg's Eggo Frozen Assorted Waffles	45g	140	6	2	0	10	240	19
Kellogg's Eggo Frozen Blueberry Muffins	46g	140	5	1.5	0	15	280	21
Kellogg's Eggo Frozen Blueberry Waffles	70g	190	6	1.5	0	15	370	29
Kellogg's Eggo Frozen Buttermilk Waffles	70g	180	6	2	0	15	420	26
Kellogg's Eggo Frozen Chocolate Chip Muffins	46g	140	5	1.5	0	15	270	21
Kellogg's Eggo Frozen Chocolate Chip Waffles	70g	210	7	2.5	0	15	380	32
Kellogg's Eggo Frozen Cinnamon Toast Waffles	92g	300	11	3	0	20	490	45
Kellogg's Eggo Frozen Homestyle Waffles	70g	190	7	2	0	20	430	27
Kellogg's Eggo Frozen Pancake Breakfast Entrée	116g	280	9	1.5	0	15	580	44
Kellogg's Eggo Frozen Strawberry Waffles	70g	190	6	1.5	0	15	370	29
Kellogg's Eggo Frozen Waffles	70g	190	7	2	0	20	430	27
Kellogg's Eggo Minis Frozen Pancake Breakfast Entrée	110g	260	8	1	0	10	550	42
Kellogg's Eggo Minis Frozen Waffles	93g	260	10	2.5	0	25	610	38
Kellogg's Nutri-Grain Eggo Frozen Blueberry Waffles	70g	180	5	1.5	0	0	380	31
Kellogg's Nutri-Grain Eggo Frozen Cinnamon Waffles	70g	170	5	1.5	0	0	310	31

Frozen Foods

	Serving	Calories	Total fat (gm)	Saturated fat (gm)	Trans fats (gm)	Cholesterol (mg)	Sodium (mg)	Carbs (gm)
Kellogg's Nutri-Grain Eggo Frozen Whole Wheat Waffles	70g	140	2.5	0.5	0	0	410	27
Kellogg's Special K Frozen Waffles	70g	160	2.5	0.5	0	20	440	29
Kemps Vanilla Ice Cream	64g	120	5	3.5	0	25	40	16
Kid Cuisine Frozen Chicken Breast & Rib Meat Entrée	245g	420	13	3	0	20	760	62
Kid Cuisine Frozen Chicken Nuggets Macaroni, Corn & Dessert Entrée	249g	400	15	4	0	30	580	51
Kid Cuisine Frozen Chicken Nuggets, Corn & Dessert Entrée	227g	410	15	3.5	0	30	600	51
Kid Cuisine Frozen Fish, Macaroni & Cheese, Vegetable & Dessert Entrée	215g	390	12	2.5	0	20	500	55
Kid Cuisine Frozen Fried Chicken, Potato & Vegetable Entrée	286g	470	20	5	1	95	710	48
Kid Cuisine Frozen Macaroni & Cheese, Vegetable & Dessert Entrée	301g	410	9	4	0	15	590	69
Klondike Chocolate Ice Cream Bars	81g	250	17	13	0	20	60	22
Klondike Vanilla Bars	80g	250	17	13	0	20	55	22
Klondike Heath English Toffee Ice Cream Bars	74g	240	15	11	0	10	80	24
Klondike Oreo Vanilla Oreo Cookie Ice Cream Bars	73g	260	17	11	0	15	120	26
Klondike Reese's Peanut Butter Ice Cream Bars	76g	260	16	10	0	10	95	26
Klondike Slim-A-Bear English Toffee & French Vanilla Ice Cream Bars	38g	100	6	4.5	0	5	30	12
Klondike Slim-A-Bear Vanilla & Chocolate Ice Cream Bars	46g	100	1.5	1	0	0	65	21
Klondike Slim-A-Bear Vanilla Ice Cream Bars	39g	100	6	5	0	5	20	11
Kraft Bagel-Fuls Frozen Cinnamon Bagels	71g	200	4	2.5	0	10	190	34
Kraft Bagel-Fuls Frozen Strawberry Cream Cheese Bagels	71g	200	4	2	0	10	190	34
Krusteaz Frozen Pancake Breakfast Entrée	108g	220	2.5	0.5	0	0	580	43
Le Sueur Frozen Sweet Peas	113g	80	1.5	1	0	5	440	14
Lean Pockets Frozen Chicken Cheddar Broccoli Pockets	127g	250	6	3	0	20	430	39
Lean Pockets Frozen Chicken Fajita Pockets	127g	240	7	3	0	20	660	35
Lean Pockets Frozen Chicken Parmesan Pockets	127g	290	7	3	0	25	470	45
Lean Pockets Frozen Ham & Cheddar Pockets	127g	270	8	4	0	30	540	40
Lean Pockets Frozen Philly Steak & Cheese Pockets	127g	270	7	3.5	0	25	640	39
Lean Pockets Frozen Sausage, Egg & Cheese Breakfast Sandwiches	127g	280	8	3.5	0	55	430	40

Frozen Foods

	Serving	Calories	Total fat (gm)	Saturated fat (gm)	Trans fats (gm)	Cholesterol (mg)	Sodium (mg)	Carbs (gm)
Lean Pockets Frozen Turkey, Broccoli & Cheese Pockets	127g	260	8	3.5	0	30	450	39
Lender's Frozen Plain Bagels	57g	140	0.5	0	0	0	300	29
Luigi's Frozen Italian Ice	171ml	130	0	0	0	0	15	32
M & M's Vanilla Ice Cream Bars	49g	190	15	12	0	10	30	13
M & M's Vanilla Ice Cream Sandwiches	66g	220	10	5	0	25	150	29
Mama Lucia Frozen Meatballs	90g	210	14	5	0.5	45	550	7
Marie Callender's Complete Dinners Frozen Chicken Fried Steak, Potato & Vegetable Entrée	425g	540	28	11	1	45	1510	51
Marie Callender's Complete Dinners Frozen Chicken, Mashed Potato & Green Been Entrée	397g	340	12	3.5	0	50	1130	38
Marie Callender's Complete Dinners Frozen Chicken, Vegetable & Pasta Entrée	397g	570	13	1.5	0	20	770	97
Marie Callender's Complete Dinners Frozen Country Fried Chicken, Mashed Potatoe & Corn Entrée	454g	560	26	8	0	60	1590	61
Marie Callender's Complete Dinners Frozen Country Fried Pork Chop, Mashed Potato & Vegetable Entrée	425g	530	25	7	0	60	1600	52
Marie Callender's Complete Dinners Frozen Meatloaf, Mashed Potato & Vegetable Entrée	397g	460	19	7	0	55	1120	40
Marie Callender's Complete Dinners Frozen Roast Beef, Mashed Potato & Vegetable Entrée	411g	340	11	4	0	45	1360	38
Marie Callender's Complete Dinners Frozen Roast Chicken, Potato & Vegetable Entrée	397g	460	25	7	0	65	1030	26
Marie Callender's Complete Dinners Frozen Salisbury Steak, Vegetable & Macaroni & Cheese Entrée	397g	390	15	5	0	60	930	38
Marie Callender's Complete Dinners Frozen Turkey, Vegetable, Potato & Stuffing Entrée	397g	350	10	2.5	0	40	1340	41
Marie Callender's Frozen Banana Cream Pie	107g	290	17	8	2	40	210	30
Marie Callender's Frozen Beef Lasagna Entrée	227g	260	10	5	0	35	960	32
Marie Callender's Frozen Beef Pot Pie	234g	510	29	11	0	30	780	47
Marie Callender's Frozen Cheesy Chicken & Vegetable & Rice Entrée	397g	460	18	10	0	75	1450	45
Marie Callender's Frozen Chicken Pot Pie	234g	520	31	12	0	25	880	45
Marie Callender's Frozen Chocolate Satin Pie	99g	410	29	14	4.5	50	200	36
Marie Callender's Frozen Coconut Cream Pie	107g	310	18	10	2	35	220	32

rozen Foods

Food	Serving	Calories	Total fat (gm)	Saturated fat (gm)	Trans fats (gm)	Cholesterol (mg)	Sodium (mg)	Carbs (gm)
Marie Callender's Frozen Creamy Chicken hrimp Linguine Entrée	369g	420	15	7	0	60	1200	45
Marie Callender's Frozen Creamy Mushroom Chicken Pot Pie	234g	540	33	13	0	20	780	48
Marie Callender's Frozen Dutch Apple Pie	128g	320	15	3.5	4	0	170	47
Marie Callender's Frozen Lemon Meringue ie	110g	260	9	2.5	2	40	190	44
Marie Callender's Frozen Razzleberry Pie	126g	360	18	4	4.5	0	300	47
Marie Callender's Frozen Shrimp Scampi Linguine Entrée	369g	380	15	8	0	70	1200	45
Marie Callender's Frozen Turkey Pot Pie	234g	510	29	11	0	20	870	46
Marie Callender's Frozen White Chicken ot Pie	284g	640	38	14	0	30	1100	56
Marie Callender's One-Dish Classics rozen Chicken & Fettucine Entrée	369g	650	40	16	1	70	1150	41
Marie Callender's One-Dish Classics rozen Chicken Alfredo Bake Entrée	369g	640	39	15	0.5	80	1230	43
McCain Ellio's Frozen Crust Cheese Pizza	138g	290	6	3	0	15	530	43
McCain Ellio's Frozen Crust Pepperoni izza	137g	310	10	4.5	0	20	620	40
McCain Frozen Sweet Potato French Fries	85g	120	3	0.5	0	0	180	22
McCain Smiles Frozen Potato Puffs	85g	160	6	1	0	0	390	24
Michelina's Frozen Chicken Fettucine & roccoli Entrée	241g	310	10	6	0	45	690	38
Michelina's Lean Gourmet Frozen Chicken ettucine & Vegetable Entrée	227g	250	7	3.5	0	40	690	34
Morningstar Farms Chicken Nuggets	86g	190	9	1.5	0	0	600	19
Morningstar Farms Frozen Hot & Spicy oultry Substitute	85g	200	8	1	0	0	640	20
Morningstar Farms Frozen Vegetable Meat ubstitute Breakfast Sausage Patties	38g	80	3	0.5	0	0	260	3
Morningstar Farms Frozen Vegetable Meat ubstitute Burgers	67g	120	4	0.5	0	0	350	13
Morningstar Farms Frozen Vegetable Meat ubstitute Links	45g	80	3	0.5	0	0	300	3
Morningstar Farms Frozen Vegetable Meat ubstitute Patties	67g	110	3.5	0.5	0	0	350	9
Morningstar Farms Frozen Vegetable Meat ubstitute Strips	17g	60	4.5	0.5	0	0	220	2
Morningstar Farms Meal Starters Frozen eggie Chicken Poultry Substitute	85g	140	3.5	0.5	0	0	510	6
Morningstar Farms Grillers Frozen egetable Meat Substitute Burgers	64g	130	6	1	0	0	260	5
Morningstar Farms Grillers Frozen egetable Meat Substitute Crumble	55g	80	2.5	0	0	0	240	4
Morningstar Farms Grillers Prime Frozen egetable Meat Substitute Patties	71g	170	9	1	0	0	360	4

Frozen Foods

	Serving	Calories	Total fat (gm)	Saturated fat (gm)	Trans fats (gm)	Cholesterol (mg)	Sodium (mg)	Carbs (gm)
Mr. Dells Frozen Hashbrowns	85g	60	0	0	0	0	0	12
Mrs. Smith's Frozen Cherry Pie	127g	330	16	7	0	0	300	43
Mrs. Smith's Frozen Dutch Apple Crumb Pie	127g	360	17	7	0	0	200	49
Mrs. Smith's Frozen Pumpkin Pie	127g	280	14	6	0	45	310	36
Mrs. T's Frozen Potato & Onion Pierogi	114g	160	2	0	0	5	390	32
Nestle Flintstone's Frozen Sherbet	54g	70	1	0	0	3	15	16
Nestle Vanilla Fudge Ice Cream Sundae Drumsticks	98g	340	19	10	0	20	100	36
Nestle Vanilla Ice Cream Drumsticks	96g	320	17	11	1	20	110	38
New York Frozen 5 Cheese Texas Toast	48g	180	9	2.5	0	5	350	20
New York Frozen Mozzarella & Provolone Texas Toast	48g	170	10	3	0	5	360	16
New York Frozen Garlic Breadsticks	50g	170	6	1.5	0	0	300	24
New York Frozen Garlic Texas Toast	40g	150	9	2	0	0	260	15
New York Pizzeria Dip'N Sticks Frozen Cheese & Garlic Breadsticks	72g	160	6	2	0	5	420	21
New York Pizzeria Dip'N Sticks Frozen Original Breadsticks	76g	140	4.5	1	0	0	430	21
On Cor Classics Frozen Chicken Parmigiana Entrée	132g	220	13	4	0	25	650	16
On Cor Classics Frozen Lasagna Entrée	191g	220	9	4	0.5	15	800	26
On Cor Traditionals Frozen Turkey Entrée	123g	70	3.5	1	0	20	790	6
Ore Ida ABC Frozen Alphabet Shaped Tater Tots	76g	160	8	1.5	0	0	410	22
Ore Ida Crispers Frozen French Fries	84g	220	13	2.5	0	0	390	23
Ore Ida Crispy Crowns Frozen Seasoned Cut Potatoes	89g	170	10	2	0	0	490	21
Ore Ida Crispy Crunchies Frozen Steak French Fries	81g	150	7	1	0	0	310	21
Ore Ida Fast Food Fries	84g	160	6	1	0	0	440	23
Ore Ida Frozen French Fries	84g	180	8	1.5	0	0	450	25
Ore Ida Frozen Hashbrowns	89g	80	0	0	0	0	55	18
Ore Ida Frozen Onion Rings	76g	170	9	1.5	0	0	530	23
Ore Ida Frozen Onion Tater Tots	90g	170	8	1.5	0	0	350	23
Ore Ida Frozen Original Potatoes	81g	130	5	1	0	0	380	18
Ore Ida Frozen Seasoned Country Fries	283g	130	4.5	1	0	0	300	20
Ore Ida Frozen Seasoned French Fries	84g	150	6	1	0	0	450	22
Ore Ida Frozen Tater Tots	95g	170	8	1.5	0	0	420	20
Ore Ida Onion Ringers Frozen Onion Rings	120g	180	10	1.5	0	0	150	21
Ore Ida Steam N' Mash Frozen Russet Potatoes Side Dish	95g	80	0	0	0	0	260	17

rozen Foods

	Serving	Calories	Total fat (gm)	Saturated fat (gm)	Trans fats (gm)	Cholesterol (mg)	Sodium (mg)	Carbs (gm)
Ore Ida Steam N' Mash Frozen Garlic Seasoned Potatoes Side Dish	131g	110	4	2.5	0	10	330	17
Ore Ida Texas Crispers Frozen Hot & Spicy Potato Wedges	84g	150	6	1	0	0	230	21
Ore Ida Zesties Frozen Seasoned French Fries	84g	150	5	1	0	0	320	22
Ore Ida Golden Crinkles Frozen French Fries	84g	120	3.5	2	0	0	310	20
Ore Ida Golden Twirls Curly Frozen French Fries	84g	160	6	1	0	0	400	24
Palermo's Primo Thin Frozen Ultra Thin Family Pepperoni Pizza	148g	380	23	11	0	60	1000	24
Pepperidge Farm Frozen 5 Cheeses & Garlic Bread	56g	210	11	4.5	0	5	320	21
Pepperidge Farm Frozen Chocolate Fudge Three Layer Cake	69g	230	10	2.5	1.5	20	130	33
Pepperidge Farm Frozen Coconut Three Layer Cake	69g	240	10	3	1.5	20	120	35
Pepperidge Farm Frozen Lemon Cake	69g	240	11	2.5	3	25	130	34
Pepperidge Farm Frozen Mozzarella Monterey Jack Texas Toast	45g	180	9	2	0	5	250	20
Pepperidge Farm Frozen Pastries	89g	270	15	8	0	0	370	31
Pepperidge Farm Frozen Puff Pastries	41g	170	11	6	0	0	270	14
Pepperidge Farm Frozen Garlic Bread	50g	180	8	3	0	0	270	21
Pepperidge Farm Frozen Garlic Texas Toast	40g	140	7	2.5	0	0	210	15
Perdue Frozen Bourbon Chicken	84g	180	8	3	0	25	360	17
Perdue Frozen Sweet & Spicy Chicken	85g	180	8	3	0	25	660	12
Philly Gourmet Frozen Beef Patties	73g	240	18	7	0	50	40	0
Pillsbury Frozen Butter Biscuits	59g	170	8	2	3.5	0	560	22
Pillsbury Frozen Crusty French Dinner Rolls	35g	80	1	0	0	0	160	16
Pillsbury Frozen Pancake Breakfast Entrée	116g	240	4	0.5	0	10	400	47
Pillsbury Home Baked Classics Frozen Buttermilk Biscuits	59g	180	8	2	3.5	0	56	22
Pillsbury Ritz Deep Dish Frozen Pie Crust	21g	90	5	2	0	5	85	11
Pillsbury Savorings Frozen Cheese & Spinach Appetizer	80g	260	17	8	0	25	430	20
Pillsbury Savorings Frozen Pepperoni & Mozarella Cheese Appetizer	80g	250	16	7	0	20	450	21
Pillsbury Toaster Scrambles Frozen Toaster Pastry Breakfast Sandwich	47g	180	11	3.5	0.5	20	300	16
Pillsbury Toaster Strudel Frozen Toaster Pastries	54g	200	11	4.5	1.5	10	220	23
Poppers Frozen Cheddar Cheese Stuffed Jalapeno Pepper	76g	190	11	4	0	15	680	19
Poppers Frozen Cream Cheese Stuffed Jalapeno Pepper	77g	220	15	6	0	25	470	18

Frozen Foods

Frozen Foods	Serving	Calories	Total fat (gm)	Saturated fat (gm)	Trans fats (gm)	Cholesterol (mg)	Sodium (mg)	Carbs (gm)
Popsicle Dora The Explorer Frozen Popsicles	70g	60	0	0	0	0	10	14
Popsicle Firecracker Frozen Fruit Juice Bars	45g	35	0	0	0	0	0	9
Popsicle Firecracker Super Heroes Frozen Fruit Juice Bars	51g	40	0	0	0	0	5	10
Popsicle Frozen Fruit Juice Bars	53g	45	0	0	0	0	0	11
Popsicle Frozen Ice Drinks	51g	15	0	0	0	0	0	4
Popsicle Mighty Magic Frozen Fruit Juice Bars	48g	40	0	0	0	0	0	9
Popsicle Scribblers Frozen Fruit Juice Bars	77g	60	0	0	0	0	10	15
Purnell Old Folks Frozen Whole Hog Breakfast Sausages	56g	220	19	6	0	50	300	0
Reames Frozen Egg Noodles	60g	170	2	0.5	0	70	10	32
Red Baron Frozen 5 Cheese & Garlic French Bread	126g	410	22	8	0	25	880	39
Red Baron Frozen Classic Crust 4 Cheese Pizza	146g	380	16	9	0.5	30	690	40
Red Baron Frozen Classic Crust Four Meat Pizza	149g	380	16	8	0	30	770	41
Red Baron Frozen Classic Crust Pepperoni Pizza	142g	370	16	8	0	30	740	40
Red Baron Frozen Classic Crust Sausage & Pepperoni Pizza	150g	400	19	9	0	35	770	41
Red Baron Frozen Classic Crust Special Deluxe Pizza	157g	380	18	8	0	30	720	41
Red Baron Frozen Classic Crust Supreme Pizza	128g	310	14	7	0	25	590	33
Red Baron Frozen Pepperoni French Bread	153g	360	15	7	0	30	1070	42
Red Baron Frozen Supreme French Bread	164g	360	15	7	0	30	1010	42
Red Baron Pizzeria Style Frozen Thin Crust Five Cheese Pizza	150g	390	17	9	0.5	30	810	42
Red Baron Pizzeria Style Frozen Thin Crust Pepperoni Pizza	149g	410	20	9	0.5	35	970	40
Red Baron Singles Frozen Deep Dish Cheese Pizza	159g	400	16	8	0	25	730	45
Red Baron Singles Frozen Deep Dish Meat Trio Pizza	159g	400	18	8	0	25	790	45
Red Baron Singles Frozen Deep Dish Pepperoni Pizza	159g	420	19	9	0	25	870	45
Red Baron Singles Frozen Deep Dish Supreme Pizza	163g	420	19	9	0	30	770	45
Red Baron Stone Hearth Frozen Fire Baked Crust Pepperoni Pizza	141g	370	17	6	0.5	30	910	39
Red Baron Super Singles Frozen Deep Dish Four Cheese Pizza	159g	410	18	10	0	30	760	45
Redi Serve Frozen Chicken Nibblers	77g	250	16	4	0	35	600	14

Frozen Foods

	Serving	Calories	Total fat (gm)	Saturated fat (gm)	Trans fats (gm)	Cholesterol (mg)	Sodium (mg)	Carbs (gm)
Rhodes Frozen White Dinner Rolls	38g	100	1.5	0	0	0	130	19
Rosetto Frozen Cheese Ravioli	131g	230	4	2	0	15	290	37
Sara Lee Frozen Apple Pie	131g	340	16	7	0	0	330	47
Sara Lee Frozen Cherry Pie	131g	340	16	7	0	0	350	45
Sara Lee Frozen Dutch Apple Pie	131g	340	14	6	0	0	290	52
Sara Lee Frozen Plain Cheesecake	121g	330	17	8	1.5	70	260	35
Sara Lee Frozen Pumpkin Pie	131g	260	10	4	0	40	320	39
Sara Lee Frozen Strawberry Cheesecake	123g	320	18	10	2	15	180	37
Seapak Frozen Breaded Butterfly Shrimp	84g	210	10	1.5	0	60	480	20
Seapak Frozen Breaded Shrimp	84g	210	10	1.5	0	60	480	20
Seapak Frozen Shrimp	113g	320	30	12	0	110	760	4
Simply Potatoes Onion & Potato Side Dish	87g	80	0	0	0	0	170	19
Simply Potatoes Potato Side Dish	124g	120	6	4	0	20	420	15
Simply Potatoes Southwestern Potato Side Dish	80g	80	0	0	0	0	240	17
Sister Schubert's Frozen Yeast Dinner Rolls	43g	140	4	1	0	10	230	23
Snickers Frozen Ice Cream Bars	50g	180	11	6	0	15	60	18
State Fair Frozen Beef Corndogs	76g	220	10	3.5	0	20	540	25
State Fair Frozen Pork & Turkey Corndogs	76g	220	12	3.5	0	25	540	22
Steak Umm Frozen Beef Sandwich	32g	100	9	3.5	0	25	20	0
Stouffer's Corner Bistro Frozen Philly Steak & Cheese Panini	170g	340	16	6	0	40	680	33
Stouffer's Corner Bistro Frozen Smoked Turkey Club Panini	170g	360	16	7	0	55	920	31
Stouffer's Corner Bistro Frozen Southwestern Chicken Panini	170g	360	16	7	0	45	920	31
Stouffer's Corner Bistro Frozen Grilled Chicken Panini	170g	350	17	6	0	35	610	31
Stouffer's Easy Express Frozen Manicotti Entrée	279g	340	16	8	0	45	950	33
Stouffer's Easy Express Frozen Rigatoni with Chicken Entrée	140g	260	10	2.5	0	20	430	29
Stouffer's Frozen Barbecue Chicken Tenders, Potato with Bacon Entrée	283g	440	19	6	0	70	1290	44
Stouffer's Frozen Beef & Macaroni Entrée	365g	410	16	7	1	40	990	45
Stouffer's Frozen Beef & Ricotta Cheese Lasagna Entrée	215g	260	9	4.5	0	30	700	28
Stouffer's Frozen Beef Lasagna Bake Entrée	326g	350	10	4	0.5	30	960	49
Stouffer's Frozen Bourbon Beefsteak & Mashed Potatoes Entrée	396g	580	24	6	0	45	1160	68
Stouffer's Frozen Broccoli & Chicken Pasta Bake Entrée	236g	300	14	6	0.5	45	990	24
Stouffer's Frozen Chicken & Mashed Potatoes Entrée	251g	250	10	3	0	60	730	20

Frozen Foods

	Serving	Calories	Total fat (gm)	Saturated fat (gm)	Trans fats (gm)	Cholesterol (mg)	Sodium (mg)	Carbs (gm)
Stouffer's Frozen Chicken Alfredo Entrée	233g	320	16	4.5	0	30	890	28
Stouffer's Frozen Chicken Enchilada, Rice & Vegetable Entrée	201g	280	12	7	0.5	40	720	30
Stouffer's Frozen Chicken Fettucine & Broccoli Entrée	297g	570	27	7	0	50	850	55
Stouffer's Frozen Chicken Lasagna Entrée	221g	320	16	4.5	0	25	790	31
Stouffer's Frozen Chicken Pot Pie	283g	660	37	14	0.5	50	1060	62
Stouffer's Frozen Chicken, Vegetable & Rice Bake Entrée	236g	360	15	6	0	70	880	37
Stouffer's Frozen Chicken, Vegetable & Rice Entrée	326g	360	12	4	0	35	800	44
Stouffer's Frozen Cream Chipped Beef Entrée	125g	140	7	4	0	35	590	11
Stouffer's Frozen Deluxe French Bread For Two	175g	430	21	7	0	25	820	44
Stouffer's Frozen Extra Cheese French Bread For Two	167g	400	18	7	0	25	630	44
Stouffer's Frozen Five Cheese Lasagna Entrée	304g	370	14	7	0	35	960	39
Stouffer's Frozen Homestyle Beef, Potato, & Vegetable Entrée	354g	300	11	3	0	40	1390	32
Stouffer's Frozen Italian Lasagna Entrée	213g	340	12	7	0	35	650	42
Stouffer's Frozen Lasagna Entrée	245g	300	12	6	0	35	850	35
Stouffer's Frozen Macaroni & Cheese Broccoli Entrée	340g	480	20	8	0.5	35	1000	52
Stouffer's Frozen Macaroni & Cheese Entrée	225g	350	17	7	0	25	920	34
Stouffer's Frozen Meat Lasagna Entrée	297g	350	11	6	0.5	40	930	38
Stouffer's Frozen Meatball & Pasta Entrée	326g	560	27	12	1	100	1250	47
Stouffer's Frozen Meatloaf & Mashed Pototo Entrée	453g	600	31	12	1.5	90	1310	45
Stouffer's Frozen Meatloaf Entrée	156g	200	11	5	0.5	30	650	8
Stouffer's Frozen Pepperoni French Bread For Two	159g	410	20	7	0	25	810	43
Stouffer's Frozen Rigatoni with Chicken Entrée	237g	390	15	5	0	40	820	44
Stouffer's Frozen Sausage Pepperoni French Bread For Two	177g	460	24	8	0	30	880	43
Stouffer's Frozen Scalloped Chicken & Noodles Entrée	340g	450	22	4	0	65	940	43
Stouffer's Frozen Spaghetti & Meatball Entrée	357g	360	12	3.5	0	35	850	45
Stouffer's Frozen Stuffed Green Pepper Entrée	220g	150	5	1.5	0	15	780	17
Stouffer's Frozen Three Meat French Bread For Two	177g	470	25	9	0	40	990	43

Frozen Foods

	Serving	Calories	Total fat (gm)	Saturated fat (gm)	Trans fats (gm)	Cholesterol (mg)	Sodium (mg)	Carbs (gm)
Stouffer's Frozen Tuna Noodle Caserole Entrée	340g	450	20	6	0	70	990	45
Stouffer's Frozen Turkey Tetrazzini Entrée	340g	450	23	9	0	70	980	38
Stouffer's Frozen Vegetable Lasagna Entrée	297g	390	18	7	0	25	730	40
Stouffer's Frozen Garlic Chicken, Vegetables & Pasta Entrée	320g	320	6	2.5	0	40	1440	42
Stouffer's Frozen Green Peppersteak & Rice Entrée	297g	240	4	1.5	0	30	910	32
Stouffer's Large Classics Frozen Five Cheese Lasagna Entrée	237g	330	14	8	0	35	870	33
Stouffer's Lean Cuisine Cafe Classics Frozen Beef Steak, Mushrooms & Broccoli Entrée	212g	180	7	2	0	30	620	13
Stouffer's Lean Cuisine Cafe Classics Frozen Chicken & Linguine Entrée	255g	310	8	2	0	30	680	36
Stouffer's Lean Cuisine Cafe Classics Frozen Chicken & Pasta Entrée	240g	290	7	2	0	30	420	36
Stouffer's Lean Cuisine Cafe Classics Frozen Chicken Tenderloins	283g	300	3	0.5	0	30	560	51
Stouffer's Lean Cuisine Cafe Classics Frozen Chicken Tenders	251g	180	7	2.5	0	40	650	9
Stouffer's Lean Cuisine Cafe Classics Frozen Chicken, Bean & Rice Entrée	240g	260	6	3	0	45	600	33
Stouffer's Lean Cuisine Cafe Classics Frozen Chicken, Pasta, & Broccoli Entrée	255g	240	7	2	0	30	690	25
Stouffer's Lean Cuisine Cafe Classics Frozen Chicken, Vegetable & Vermicelli Entrée	297g	240	5	2	0	30	640	29
Stouffer's Lean Cuisine Cafe Classics Frozen Chicken/Almond Rice Entrée	240g	250	4	0.5	0	30	490	38
Stouffer's Lean Cuisine Cafe Classics Frozen Crisp Crust Individual Pizza	170g	340	8	2.5	0	20	510	49
Stouffer's Lean Cuisine Cafe Classics Frozen Fish & Rice Entrée	255g	330	8	2.5	0	40	590	50
Stouffer's Lean Cuisine Cafe Classics Frozen Fish, Vegetable & Rice Entrée	226g	330	9	2.5	0	35	540	45
Stouffer's Lean Cuisine Cafe Classics Frozen Salisbury Steak & Macaroni Entrée	269g	280	9	4.5	0	50	610	25
Stouffer's Lean Cuisine Cafe Classics Frozen Shrimp & Pasta Entrée	283g	220	4	1	0	50	590	32
Stouffer's Lean Cuisine Cafe Classics Frozen Shrimp Linguini & Vegetable Entrée	255g	260	5	2	0	60	590	36
Stouffer's Lean Cuisine Cafe Classics Frozen Glazed Chicken, Vegetables & Rice Entrée	240g	220	3.5	1	0	40	500	25
Stouffer's Lean Cuisine Casual Eating Classics Frozen Chicken Club Panini	170g	350	9	3.5	0	35	830	44
Stouffer's Lean Cuisine Casual Eating Classics Frozen Chicken Tuscan Panini	170g	320	7	2	0	25	590	41

Frozen Foods

Frozen Foods	Serving	Calories	Total fat (gm)	Saturated fat (gm)	Trans fats (gm)	Cholesterol (mg)	Sodium (mg)	Carbs (gm)
Stouffer's Lean Cuisine Casual Eating Classics Frozen Chicken, Spinach & Mushroom Panini	170g	320	7	2.5	0	30	660	41
Stouffer's Lean Cuisine Casual Eating Classics Frozen Crisp Crust Single Pizza	170g	310	5	1.5	0	5	530	52
Stouffer's Lean Cuisine Casual Eating Classics Frozen Deep Dish Single Pizza	180g	370	9	3.5	0	25	630	51
Stouffer's Lean Cuisine Casual Eating Classics Frozen Thin Crust Single Pizza	170g	320	7	3	0	5	660	49
Stouffer's Lean Cuisine Comfort Classics Frozen Beef, Mashed Potatoes & Vegetables Entrée	255g	210	6	2	0	25	550	26
Stouffer's Lean Cuisine Comfort Classics Frozen Chicken & Spaghetti Entrée	308g	310	8	2	0	35	660	39
Stouffer's Lean Cuisine Comfort Classics Frozen Chicken, Potato & Vegetable Entrée	226g	180	3.5	1	0	35	540	20
Stouffer's Lean Cuisine Comfort Classics Frozen Turkey & Vegetable Entrée	226g	150	5	1	0	25	650	12
Stouffer's Lean Cuisine Dinnertime Select Frozen Beef Tip, Potato & Vegetable Entrée	340g	280	7	2.5	0	30	650	33
Stouffer's Lean Cuisine Dinnertime Select Frozen Penne Pasta & Vegetable Entrée	340g	330	4.5	1.5	0	40	580	52
Stouffer's Lean Cuisine Dinnertime Selects Frozen Turkey Breast Dinner	340g	290	7	1	0	30	890	38
Stouffer's Lean Cuisine Everyday Favorite Frozen Chicken Fettucini Entrée	262g	270	6	3	0	40	690	32
Stouffer's Lean Cuisine Everyday Favorite Frozen Fettuccine Alfredo Entrée	262g	330	7	3	0	15	600	54
Stouffer's Lean Cuisine Everyday Favorite Frozen Meatball & Pasta Entrée	258g	300	8	3	0	45	620	34
Stouffer's Lean Cuisine Flatbread Melts Frozen Beef Steak Flatbread	177g	330	9	4	0	30	570	40
Stouffer's Lean Cuisine Flatbread Melts Frozen Chicken Flatbread	191g	330	8	3	0	20	630	43
Stouffer's Lean Cuisine Frozen Deep Dish Individual Margherita Pizza	170g	340	9	2.5	0	5	540	50
Stouffer's Lean Cuisine Frozen Deep Dish Individual Pizza	173g	330	7	4	0	10	440	51
Stouffer's Lean Cuisine Frozen Tuscan Chicken Dinner	340g	280	6	2	0	40	780	34
Stouffer's Lean Cuisine One Dish Favorite Frozen Beans & Rice Entrée	294g	300	5	2.5	0	15	590	52
Stouffer's Lean Cuisine One Dish Favorite Frozen Enchilada & Rice Entrée	255g	270	4	1.5	0	20	550	47
Stouffer's Lean Cuisine One Dish Favorite Frozen Lasagna Entrée	297g	320	7	3.5	0	30	590	43
Stouffer's Lean Cuisine One Dish Favorite Frozen Macaroni & Cheese Entrée	283g	290	7	4	0	20	630	41

rozen Foods

	Serving	Calories	Total fat (gm)	Saturated fat (gm)	Trans fats (gm)	Cholesterol (mg)	Sodium (mg)	Carbs (gm)
touffer's Lean Cuisine One Dish Favorite rozen Stuffed Cabbage & Mashed otatoes Entrée	269g	220	4	1.5	0	45	400	21
touffer's Lean Cuisine Spa Cuisine lassics Frozen Chicken Broccoli Entrée	280g	290	4	1	0	30	640	46
touffer's Lean Cuisine Spa Cuisine lassics Frozen Chicken, Vegetable & asta Entrée	255g	280	8	1.5	0	25	560	30
touffer's Lean Cuisine Spa Cuisine lassics Frozen Ravioli Entrée	280g	350	9	3	0	35	660	56
touffer's Lean Cuisine Spa Cuisine lassics Frozen Chicken & Brown Rice ntrée	265g	240	6	3	0	25	610	30
touffer's Lean Cuisine Spa Cuisine lassics Frozen Chicken Primavera Entrée	265g	220	5	1.5	0	25	610	24
touffer's Skillet Sensations Frozen hicken, Vegetable & Pasta Entrée	354g	410	10	4	0	50	980	48
uper Pretzel Frozen Pretzel Knot	64g	160	1	0	0	0	130	34
uper Pretzel Softstix Frozen Cheddar heese Pretzel Stick	50g	130	3	1.5	0	10	270	22
wanson Classics Frozen Fried Chicken, lashed Potato & Corn Dinner	213g	240	13	3	0	35	520	21
wanson Frozen Chicken Pot Pie	198g	380	22	8	0	35	770	34
GI Friday's Frozen Bacon & Cheddar tuffed Potato	96g	210	12	4	0	20	480	17
GI Friday's Frozen Chicken Quesadilla	128g	290	13	7	0.5	40	610	26
GI Friday's Frozen Chicken Quesadilla olls	87g	250	12	4	1	25	410	26
GI Friday's Frozen Chicken Wings	96g	180	11	3	0	95	1030	4
GI Friday's Frozen Creamy Chicken, Penne asta & Vegetables Entrée	270g	360	14	6	0.5	55	900	34
GI Friday's Frozen Mozzarella Cheese tick Appetizer	28g	80	4.5	2	0	10	220	7
he Skinny Cow Cookies & Cream Ice ream Sandwiches	71g	150	2	1	0	3	105	31
he Skinny Cow Chocolate Fudge Ice ream Cones	75g	150	3	2	0	4	95	28
The Skinny Cow Fudge Bars	74g	100	1	0.5	0	3	45	22
The Skinny Cow Ice Cream Sandwiches	71g	140	1.5	1	0	1	100	30
The Skinny Cow Vanilla Ice Cream Cones	75g	150	3	2	0	4	85	29
The Skinny Cow Mint Ice Cream Sandwiches	71g	140	1.5	1	0	1	95	30
The Skinny Cow Vanilla Ice Cream Sandwiches	71g	140	2	0.5	0	0	95	28
Tombstone Frozen Crust Deluxe Pizza	134g	290	12	5	0	30	580	30
Tombstone Frozen Crust Extra Cheese Pizza	145g	350	15	8	0.5	40	670	36
Tombstone Frozen Crust Pepperoni Pizza	153g	390	20	8	0	45	890	36

Frozen Foods

	Serving	Calories	Total fat (gm)	Saturated fat (gm)	Trans fats (gm)	Cholesterol (mg)	Sodium (mg)	Carbs (gm)
Tombstone Frozen Crust Sausage Pepperoni Pizza	152g	370	17	7	0	40	800	37
Tombstone Frozen Crust Sausage Pizza	125g	290	13	5	0	30	600	30
Tombstone Frozen Crust Supreme Pizza	130g	300	14	6	0	30	640	31
Tombstone Frozen Pepperoni Garlic Bread	131g	370	17	6	0.5	30	670	40
Tony's Frozen Original Crust Cheese Pizza	120g	290	12	5	0	15	570	37
Tony's Frozen Original Crust Pepperoni Pizza	119g	310	14	7	0	10	620	36
Tony's Frozen Original Crust Sausage Pepperoni Pizza	130g	340	17	8	0	15	660	37
Tony's Frozen Original Crust Supreme Pizza	136g	330	16	7	0	10	630	37
Totino's Frozen Combo Sausage Pepperoni Pizza Snack Rolls	85g	210	9	2.5	1.5	5	470	24
Totino's Frozen Crisp Crust Party 3 Cheese Pizza	138g	320	16	5	3	15	720	34
Totino's Frozen Crisp Crust Party Pizza	145g	370	21	5	4	15	960	35
Totino's Frozen Pepperoni Pizza Snack Rolls	85g	210	10	2.5	1.5	10	480	24
Totino's Frozen Supreme Pizza Snack Rolls	85g	200	8	2	1.5	5	390	25
Totino's Frozen Three Meat Pizza Snack Rolls	85g	200	8	2.5	1.5	10	470	24
Totino's Frozen Triple Cheese Pizza Snack Rolls	85g	200	8	2.5	2	5	400	24
Totino's Mega Pizza Rolls Frozen Ultimate Pepperoni Pizza Snacks	93g	230	11	3	1	15	560	25
Totino's Party Pizza Frozen Crisp Crust Single Pepperoni Pizza	145g	360	20	4.5	4	10	920	34
Totino's Party Pizza Frozen Crisp Crust Single Sausage Pizza	153g	370	20	4.5	4	10	890	35
Totino's Party Pizza Frozen Crisp Crust Single Serving Cheese Pizza	139g	310	15	3.5	3.5	10	750	34
Totino's Party Pizza Frozen Crisp Crust Single Serving Classic Pizza	145g	370	20	4.5	4	15	910	35
Totino's Party Pizza Frozen Crisp Crust Three Meat Pizza	149g	350	18	4	4	10	900	34
Totino's Pizza Rolls Frozen Cheese Pizza Snack Rolls	85g	200	8	2	2	5	480	26
Tyson Anytizers Frozen Chicken Fries	90g	230	13	3	0	25	540	14
Tyson Anytizers Frozen Chicken Popcorn Bites	84g	180	9	1.5	0	30	560	11
Tyson Anytizers Frozen Chicken Wings	84g	150	7	1.5	0	30	680	8
Tyson Anytizers Frozen Honey Barbecue Chicken Wings	96g	220	15	3.5	0	110	560	1
Tyson Anytizers Frozen Hot Spicy Chicken Wings	3	220	15	3.5	0	110	560	0
Tyson Anytizers Frozen White Meat Chicken Wings	84g	150	7	1.5	0	30	680	8

Frozen Foods

	Serving	Calories	Total fat (gm)	Saturated fat (gm)	Trans fats (gm)	Cholesterol (mg)	Sodium (mg)	Carbs (gm)
Tyson Frozen Chicken Fillets	68g	150	7	1.5	0	20	370	12
Tyson Frozen Chicken Nuggets	84g	270	21	4.5	0	45	570	11
Tyson Frozen Chicken Patties	73g	180	11	2.5	0	25	390	12
Tyson Frozen Chicken Strips	101g	230	10	2	0	40	1250	21
Tyson Frozen Honey Barbecue Chicken Strips	75g	180	8	1.5	0	15	690	18
Tyson Frozen Honey Chicken Tenders	85g	220	13	3	0	35	250	13
Van De Kamps Battered Frozen Pollock	110g	240	12	3	0	40	750	19
Van De Kamps Frozen Beer Battered Alaskan Pollock	120g	240	11	3.5	0	25	750	23
Van De Kamps Frozen Breaded Alaskan Pollock	93g	220	12	4	0	20	420	20
Van De Kamps Frozen Breaded Pollock & Whiting Fish Sticks	95g	230	10	2.5	0	35	480	22
Weight Watcher's Chocolate Chip Cookie Dough Ice Cream Cups	100g	140	2.5	1.5	0	5	80	31
Weight Watcher's Chocolate Cookies & Cream Ice Cream Bars	70g	130	4.5	1.5	0	5	100	24
Weight Watcher's Chocolate Fudge Bar	76g	110	1	0.5	0	5	70	28
Weight Watcher's Chocolate Fudge Brownie Ice Cream Cups	102g	140	1.5	1	0	5	85	35
Weight Watcher's Chocolate Fudge Sundae Ice Cream Cones	73g	140	4	1.5	0	5	70	26
Weight Watcher's Coffee Ice Cream Bars	75g	90	1	0.5	0	5	55	21
Weight Watcher's Cookies & Cream Ice Cream Bars	71g	140	5	1.5	0	5	110	26
Weight Watcher's English Toffee Crunch Ice Cream Bars	80g	220	12	10	0	5	80	26
Weight Watcher's Mint Chocolate Chip Ice Cream Cups	99g	140	3.5	2.5	0	5	80	29
Weight Watcher's Smart Ones Anytime Select Frozen Fiesta Quesadillas	113g	220	5	2.5	0	10	630	32
Weight Watcher's Smart Ones Anytime Select Frozen Italiano Calzones	142g	290	6	2	0	25	620	47
Weight Watcher's Smart Ones Bistro Select Frozen Chicken & Fettucini Entrée	283g	340	6	3	0	55	680	47
Weight Watcher's Smart Ones Bistro Select Frozen Chicken Parmesan Entrée	311g	290	5	1.5	0	40	630	35
Weight Watcher's Smart Ones Bistro Select Frozen Meatloaf & Mashed Potatoes Entrée	269g	250	8	3	0	45	880	23
Weight Watcher's Smart Ones Bistro Select Frozen Salisbury Steak & Asparagus Entrée	255g	200	7	2.5	0	40	660	14
Weight Watcher's Smart Ones Frozen Angel Hair Marinara & Zucchini Entrée	283g	230	4	1	0	0	640	40
Weight Watcher's Smart Ones Frozen Baked Potato, Broccoli & Cheddar Entrée	283g	220	6	3	0	15	480	34

Frozen Foods

Frozen Foods	Serving	Calories	Total fat (gm)	Saturated fat (gm)	Trans fats (gm)	Cholesterol (mg)	Sodium (mg)	Carbs (gm)
Weight Watcher's Smart Ones Frozen Broccoli & Pasta Entrée	255g	280	6	3.5	0	10	700	44
Weight Watcher's Smart Ones Frozen Chocolate Chip Cookie Dough Ice Cream	75g	170	3	1.5	0	5	100	32
Weight Watcher's Smart Ones Frozen Macaroni & Cheese Entrée	283g	270	2	1	0	5	790	52
Weight Watcher's Smart Ones Frozen Santa Fe Bean & Rice Entrée	283g	310	7	3	0	15	660	51
Weight Watcher's Smart Ones Frozen Schezuan Chicken Noodle & Vegetable Entrée	255g	240	5	1	0	5	900	36
Weight Watcher's Smart Ones Frozen Tuna Noodle Entrée	269g	250	4.5	1.5	0	45	780	37
Weight Watcher's Smart Ones Fruit Inspirations Frozen Chicken & Rice Entrée	255g	320	8	1.5	0	20	680	48
Weight Watcher's Smart Ones Morning Express Frozen English Muffins	113g	210	5	2.5	0	15	610	27
Weight Watcher's Smart Ones Morning Express Frozen Tortillas	113g	220	6	3	0	20	710	28
Weight Watcher's Turtle Sundae Ice Cream Cups	105g	170	5	2	0	5	105	34
Weight Watcher's Vanilla Chocolate Fudge Ice Cream Cones	73g	140	4	1.5	0	5	70	27
Weight Watcher's Vanilla Ice Cream Sandwiches	70g	140	1.5	0.5	0	5	125	31
Well's Blue Bunny Bomb Pops	52g	40	0	0	0	0	5	10
Well's Blue Bunny Vanilla Ice Cream	64g	130	7	4.5	0	25	60	16
Well's Blue Bunny Vanilla Ice Cream Sandwiches	57g	140	3	1.5	0	5	170	25
White Castle Frozen Beef Cheeseburgers	104g	310	17	8	1	40	600	26
White Castle Frozen Beef Hamburgers	90g	270	13	5	1	30	370	25
Wyman's Frozen Whole Wild Blueberry Fruit	140g	60	0	0	0	0	0	18

Meats	Serving	Calories	Total fat (gm)	Saturated fat (gm)	Trans fats (gm)	Cholesterol (mg)	Sodium (mg)	Carbs (gm)
Aidell's Chicken Sausage	85g	160	11	3.5	0	95	670	3
Aidell's Pork Sausage	85g	170	12	4.5	0	50	620	1
Al Fresco Chicken Italian Sausage	85g	110	6	2	0	65	440	2
Al Fresco Chicken Sausage	85g	160	7	2	0	60	480	10
Armour Chicken & Beef	85g	160	12	3	0	80	840	0
Armour Original Vienna Sausage Links	50g	110	10	3	0	45	490	1
Ball Park Beef Franks	50g	50	0	0	0	10	470	6
Ball Park Beef, Pork & Turkey Hot Dogs	57g	180	16	6	0	45	550	4
Ball Park Singles Beef Hot Dogs	45g	150	13	6	1	25	430	3
Ball Park Turkey Franks	50g	45	0	0	0	10	420	5
Bar-S Beef, Chicken & Pork Franks	113g	330	29	9	0	110	1290	9
Bar-S Chicken, Beef & Pork Polish Sausage	84g	240	18	5	0	100	1030	9
Bar-S Chicken, Beef & Pork Sausage	84g	240	17	5	0	100	1050	9
Bar-S Tasty Dogs Chicken Franks	56g	150	12	3.5	0	65	590	5
Bar-S Turkey Franks	56g	120	9	2.5	0	50	680	4
Bob Evans Sausage	51g	150	12	4.5	0	25	310	2
Buddig Deli Cuts Sliced White Turkey Breast	56g	70	2.5	1	0	20	460	2
Bumble Bee Albacore Tuna in Water	56g	60	1	0	0	25	180	0
Bumble Bee Albacore Tuna Solid in Water	56g	70	1.5	0	0	25	250	0
Bumble Bee Crab Seafood Meat	56g	40	1	0	0	50	300	0
Bumble Bee Pink Salmon	63g	90	5	1	0	40	270	0
Bumble Bee Prime Fillet Albacore Tuna Solid in Water	56g	70	1	0	0	25	180	0
Bumble Bee Sockeye Red Salmon	63g	110	7	1.5	0	40	270	0
Bumble Bee Tuna in Oil	56g	70	3	0.5	0	25	180	0
Bumble Bee Tuna in Water	56g	50	0.5	0	0	30	180	0
Butterball Natural Smoked Bacon	14g	25	1.5	0.5	0	10	135	0
Butterball Thin Smoked Bacon	27g	50	3.5	1	0	20	260	1
Chicken of The Sea Albacore Tuna Solid in Water	56g	70	1	0	0	25	250	0
Chicken of The Sea Pink Salmon	63g	90	5	1	0	40	270	0
Chicken of The Sea Tuna in Oil	56g	100	6	1	0	25	250	0
Chicken of The Sea Tuna in Spring Water	56g	60	0.5	0	0	30	250	0
Chicken of The Sea Tuna in Water	56g	50	0.5	0	0	25	250	0
Corn King Smoked Bacon	15g	90	7	2.5	0	15	270	0
Curly's Hickory Smoked BBQ Pork Entrée	59g	110	4	1.5	0	20	450	10
Eckrich Pork, Turkey & Beef Sausage	56g	180	15	6	0	35	490	4
Eckrich Turkey & Pork Franks	45g	140	12	4	0	20	450	4
Farmland Chicken, Pork & Beef Frankfurters	57g	170	14	4.5	0	55	650	4

Meats

Meats	Serving	Calories	Total fat (gm)	Saturated fat (gm)	Trans fats (gm)	Cholesterol (mg)	Sodium (mg)	Carbs (gm)
Farmland Hickory Smoked Bacon	15g	80	7	3	0	15	260	0
Hatfield Ham	84g	90	1.5	0.5	0	20	700	2
Hatfield Hardwood Smoked Bacon	14g	70	5	2	0	5	290	0
Healthy Ones Sliced Ham	56g	60	1.5	0.5	0	25	470	4
Healthy Ones Sliced White Turkey Breast	56g	60	1.5	0.5	0	25	470	3
Hebrew National Beef Franks	85g	270	26	11	1	45	720	1
Hebrew National Beef German Sausage	85g	260	24	10	1	55	810	1
Hickory Farm's Beef Summer Sausage	56g	190	16	7	1	40	770	1
Hillshire Farm's Beef Polish Sausage	58g	170	15	6	1	35	520	3
Hillshire Farm's Beef Sausage	66g	180	15	6	1	35	710	3
Hillshire Farm's Cheddarwurst Pork & Beef Sausage	76g	240	21	8	0	55	660	3
Hillshire Farm's Deli Select Hearty Thick Ham	28g	30	0.5	0	0	10	260	1
Hillshire Farm's Deli Select Hearty Thick Turkey Breast	28g	25	0	0	0	10	260	1
Hillshire Farm's Deli Select Thin Sliced Ham	57g	60	1.5	0	0	30	750	3
Hillshire Farm's Deli Select Thin Sliced Turkey Breast	57g	50	0.5	0	0	25	730	3
Hillshire Farm's Deli Select Ultra Thin Brown Sugar Ham	56g	60	1.5	0	0	30	620	3
Hillshire Farm's Deli Select Ultra Thin Chicken Breast	56g	50	0.5	0	0	30	700	2
Hillshire Farm's Deli Select Ultra Thin Ham	56g	60	1.5	0.5	0	30	670	1
Hillshire Farm's Deli Select Ultra Thin Hard Salami	28g	110	10	4	0	30	500	0
Hillshire Farm's Deli Select Ultra Thin Roast Beef	56g	70	3	1	0	30	550	1
Hillshire Farm's Deli Select Ultra Thin Turkey Breast	56g	50	0.5	0	0	20	690	1
Hillshire Farm's Little Beef Smokies Beef Sausage	50g	160	14	7	1	35	440	2
Hillshire Farm's Pork & Beef Polish Sausage	56g	190	17	6	0	35	610	3
Hillshire Farm's Pork & Beef Sausage	66g	200	16	7	0.5	40	760	3
Hillshire Farm's Pork Sausage	50g	160	15	6	0	35	490	1
Hillshire Farm's Turkey, Pork & Beef Sausage	56g	110	8	3	0	35	510	0
Honeysuckle White Turkey	112g	120	1	0	0	70	55	0
Hormel Always Tender Honey Mustard Pork	112g	140	5	2	0	45	510	4
Hormel Always Tender Mesquite Barbecue Pork	112g	120	4	1.5	0	45	550	2
Hormel Always Tender Original Pork	112g	130	5	2	0	45	360	1
Hormel Always Tender Peppercorn Pork	112g	120	4	1.5	0	50	630	2

Meats	Serving	Calories	Total fat (gm)	Saturated fat (gm)	Trans fats (gm)	Cholesterol (mg)	Sodium (mg)	Carbs (gm)
Hormel Always Tender Teriyaki Pork	112g	130	4	1.5	0	50	500	5
Hormel Always Tender Garlic & Lemon Pork	112g	130	5	2	0	45	600	1
Hormel Beef Entrée	140g	170	8	3.5	0.5	60	700	5
Hormel Beef Meatloaf Entrée	140g	260	13	7	0.5	60	870	13
Hormel Black Label Center Cut Bacon	14g	70	5	2	0	15	300	0
Hormel Black Label Maple Bacon	15g	80	7	2.5	0	15	270	0
Hormel Black Label Original Bacon	15g	80	7	2.5	0	15	330	0
Hormel Black Label Thick Bacon	21g	110	9	3.5	0	20	460	0
Hormel Meat Corned Beef	56g	120	6	3.5	0	20	490	0
Hormel Natural Choice Deli Ham	56g	70	1.5	0.5	0	30	520	3
Hormel Natural Choice Deli Turkey	56g	50	1	0	0	25	490	1
Hormel Pork	56g	320	33	10	0	40	1200	0
Hormel Pork Roast Entrée	140g	180	7	2.5	0	85	600	1
Hormel Premium Chicken	56g	60	1.5	0.5	0	40	250	0
Hormel Roast Beef	140g	210	10	4	0	80	450	3
Hormel Smoked Bacon	15g	80	7	2.5	0	20	300	0
Hormel Spam Lite Luncheon Meat	56g	110	8	3	0	40	580	1
Hormel Spam Luncheon Meat	56g	180	16	6	0	40	790	1
Hormel Thick Canadian Bacon	56g	70	2.5	1	0	30	650	0
Hormel Turkey Breast Entrée	161g	130	3	1	0	50	1150	4
IBP Beef	112g	280	23	9	0	86	70	0
Jennie-O Smoked Bacon	15g	20	0.5	0	0	10	140	0
Jennie-O Turkey	112g	120	1.5	0.5	0	55	70	0
Jennie-O Turkey Franks	34g	70	5	1.5	0	25	370	1
Jimmy Dean Original Bacon	10g	45	4	1.5	0	10	160	0
Jimmy Dean Original Sausage	68g	260	24	8	0	50	710	2
Jimmy Dean Sage Sausage	56g	180	16	5	0	40	420	1
Jimmy Dean Sausage	68g	120	7	2	0	55	490	1
John Morrell Beef, Chicken & Pork Frankfurters	43g	150	13	4.5	0	35	550	4
John Morrell Hardwood Smoked Bacon	17g	100	9	3	0	10	300	0
John Morrell off The Bone Thick Turkey Breast	56g	80	2	0.5	0	25	390	6
Johnsonville Sausage	76g	190	16	6	0	40	610	1
Johnsonville Pork Sausage	112g	300	25	9	0	65	800	2
Jones Canadian Bacon	51g	60	1.5	0.5	0	30	460	1
Kahn's Stacked Braunschweiger Pack	56g	180	16	9	0	80	650	3
King Oscar Brisling Sardines	85g	150	11	2.5	0	120	340	0
Land O' Frost Premium Deli Thin Ham	50g	60	3	1	0	25	560	1

Meats

Meats	Serving	Calories	Total fat (gm)	Saturated fat (gm)	Trans fats (gm)	Cholesterol (mg)	Sodium (mg)	Carbs (gm)
Land O' Frost Premium Deli Thin Honey Ham	50g	70	3	1	0	25	530	2
Land O' Frost Premium Turkey Breast	52g	80	4.5	1	0	25	650	3
Libby's Corned Beef	56g	120	7	3	0	40	490	0
Libby's Vienna Sausage Link	48g	130	12	5	0	40	260	1
Lightlife Smart Dogs Meatless Hot Dogs	42g	45	0	0	0	0	310	2
Lloyd's Barbecue Beef Entrée	56g	80	2	1	0	20	360	9
Lloyd's Barbecue Chicken Entrée	56g	80	2	1	0	15	360	9
Lloyd's Barbecue Pork Baby Back Ribs	137g	290	17	7	0	70	850	20
Lloyd's Barbecue Pork Entrée	56g	80	2	1	0	15	360	9
Lloyd's Pork Spare Ribs	137g	350	24	9	0	70	750	16
Louis Rich Oscar Mayer Turkey Franks	45g	100	8	2.5	0	30	510	2
Nathan Beef Franks	57g	170	15	6	0	35	470	1
Oscar Mayer Bacon	14g	70	6	2	0	15	290	0
Oscar Mayer Beef Franks	45g	90	7	3	0	20	380	2
Oscar Mayer Beef Wiener	76g	230	22	9	1.5	50	740	1
Oscar Mayer Bologna	28g	25	0.5	0	0	10	240	3
Oscar Mayer Center Cut Bacon	34g	50	3.5	1	0	15	210	0
Oscar Mayer Centercut Thick Slice Bacon	18g	70	5	2	0	20	320	0
Oscar Mayer Cotto Salami	28g	70	6	2	0	25	280	1
Oscar Mayer Deli Fresh Shaved Ham	51g	50	1	0.5	0	25	650	2
Oscar Mayer Deli Fresh Shaved Roast Beef	51g	60	2	1	0	30	530	0
Oscar Mayer Fast Frank Beef Hot Dog Sandwich	96g	320	20	8	1	35	700	24
Oscar Mayer Hard Salami	27g	100	8	3	0	25	510	1
Oscar Mayer Hardwood Smoked Bacon	45g	70	6	2	0	15	290	0
Oscar Mayer Pegged Rigid Pack Bologna	28g	60	4	1.5	0	15	240	2
Oscar Mayer Pegged Rigid Pack Ham	64g	50	1.5	0.5	0	15	740	0
Oscar Mayer Shaved Chicken Breast	51g	50	1	0	0	25	530	2
Oscar Mayer Shaved Ham	51g	60	1	0	0	25	740	3
Oscar Mayer Stacked Rigid Pack Bologna	28g	60	4	1	0	25	220	2
Oscar Mayer Turkey & Beef Wieners	50g	40	0.5	0	0	15	470	3
Oscar Mayer Turkey, Pork & Beef Wieners	45g	90	6	2	0	30	380	1
Oscar Mayer Turkey, Pork & Chicken Wieners	45g	130	12	4	0	35	540	1
Perri Pork Italian Sausage	77g	230	20	7	0	50	540	1
Plumrose Ham	170g	150	4.5	1.5	0	50	1800	3
Plumrose Hardwood Smoked Bacon	2	110	9	3.5	0	20	410	0
Plumrose Stacked Ham	42g	50	1.5	0	0	25	450	0
Purnell Old Folks Mild Sausage	56g	220	19	6	0	50	300	0

Meats

Meats	Serving	Calories	Total fat (gm)	Saturated fat (gm)	Trans fats (gm)	Cholesterol (mg)	Sodium (mg)	Carbs (gm)
Ready Crisp Smoked Bacon	13g	70	6	2.5	0	15	270	0
Sabrett Beef Frankfurters	57g	170	15	6	0	20	530	1
Sabrett Beef Franks	57g	170	15	6	0	35	510	1
Sara Lee Fresh Ideas Ham	51g	60	1.5	0.5	0	25	550	3
Sara Lee Fresh Ideas Turkey Breast	51g	50	0.5	0	0	20	550	1
Shady Brook Farms Turkey Italian Sausage	93g	160	9	2.5	0	55	590	2
Snow's Clam Juice	15ml	0	0	0	0	0	70	0
Snow's Clam Seafood	56g	25	0	0	0	10	320	2
Starkist Albacore Tuna in Water	74g	90	2	0.5	0	30	310	1
Starkist Albacore Tuna Solid in Water	79g	110	2.5	0.5	0	40	240	1
Starkist Tuna in Vegetable Oil	56g	90	4.5	1	0	20	190	2
Starkist Tuna in Water	79g	80	1	0	0	35	250	1
Swanson Chicken Meat	56g	50	1	0	0	25	260	1
The Turkey Store Mild Breakfast Sausage	56g	140	11	3	0	45	360	0
The Turkey Store Turkey Italian Sausage	109g	160	10	2.5	0	70	890	0
Tyson Beef Entrée	140g	200	12	4.5	0	55	530	5
Tyson Beef Pot Roast	140g	170	8	3	0	65	730	2
Tyson Chicken Meat	56g	60	1	0	0	30	200	0
Tyson Oven Roasted Chicken	84g	110	2.5	1	0	65	330	2
Tyson Smoked Chicken Strips	84g	100	1.5	0.5	0	55	390	3
Tyson Thick Smoked Bacon	24g	140	11	4	0	25	380	0
Underwood Chicken Spread	56g	130	8	2	0.5	30	350	2
Underwood Deviled Ham	60g	180	15	5	0	35	480	1
Valley Fresh Chicken	56g	70	2	1	0	40	180	0

Grocery Food Factoid:

70%—The percentage of all cancers that are caused by a poor diet, lack of physical activity, and tobacco use. Most cancers are caused by the way we live our lives, not genetics or toxins.

Packaged Desserts	Serving	Calories	Total fat (gm)	Saturated fat (gm)	Trans fats (gm)	Cholesterol (mg)	Sodium (mg)	Carbs (gm)
Altoids Curiously Strong Peppermints	2g	10	0	0	0	0	0	2
Andes Chocolate Creme De Menthe Mints	38g	200	13	11	0	0	20	22
Cadbury Milk Chocolate	39g	200	11	7	0	10	40	23
Dove Dark Chocolate Miniatures	40g	210	13	8	0	5	0	24
Dove Milk Chocolate	40g	220	13	8	0	10	25	24
Drake's Devil's Food Crème Filled Devil Dogs	45g	170	7	3	0	0	125	27
Drake's Ring Dings Chocolate Snack Cakes	77g	330	17	12	0	0	230	44
Drake's Yodels Chocolate Snack Cakes	62g	270	14	9	0	10	140	37
Entenmann's Chocolate Chip Cookies	30g	140	7	3	0	5	80	20
Entenmann's Little Bites Fudge Brownies	62g	270	14	4	0	40	200	35
Good & Plenty Licorice	1 box	170	0	0	0	0	120	43
Heath Milk Chocolate English Toffee Miniatures	43g	230	14	7	0	10	150	27
Hershey's Bliss Dark Chocolate	43g	200	14	9	0	5	10	25
Hershey's Bliss Milk Chocolate	43g	210	14	9	0	5	40	24
Hershey's Kisses Milk Chocolate	41g	200	12	7	0	10	35	25
Hershey's Kisses Milk Chocolate with Almonds	40g	210	14	7	0	10	30	21
Hershey's Milk Chocolate Almond Bar	40g	210	14	7	0	10	30	21
Hershey's Milk Chocolate Bar	41g	210	14	6	0	10	25	21
Hershey's Mr. Goodbar Chocolate with Peanuts	42g	200	12	8	0	10	35	25
Hershey's Nuggets Dark Chocolate with Almonds	49g	250	17	7	0	5	65	26
Hershey's Nuggets Milk Chocolate	38g	220	14	6	0	5	0	20
Hershey's Nuggets Milk Chocolate Almond Toffee	41g	230	13	8	0	10	35	24
Hershey's Special Dark Chocolate	41g	180	12	8	0	5	15	25
Hershey's Symphony Milk Chocolate	38g	180	12	7	0	5	15	23
Hostess 100 Calorie Packs Chocolate Snack Cakes	37g	100	3	1.5	0	10	140	22
Hostess Chocolate Cupcakes	50g	180	6	3	0	5	290	31
Hostess Dessert Cups	32g	110	2	0	0	20	140	21
Hostess Twinkies Golden Snack Cakes	43g	150	4.5	2.5	0	20	220	27
Hunt's Snack Pack Flavored Pudding	99g	110	3.5	2	0	0	150	18
Jello Dark Chocolate Pudding	106g	60	1.5	1.5	0	0	170	13
Jello Double Chocolate Pudding	106g	60	1	1	0	60	170	13
Jello Strawberry Gelatin	99g	70	0	0	0	0	40	17
Jello Tapioca Pudding	113g	110	1	1	0	0	200	25
Jello Vanilla Caramel Sundae Pudding	160g	60	1	1	0	0	170	12
Jello Vanilla Pudding	113g	110	1	1	0	0	190	23

Packaged Desserts	Serving	Calories	Total fat (gm)	Saturated fat (gm)	Trans fats (gm)	Cholesterol (mg)	Sodium (mg)	Carbs (gm)
Jolly Rancher Assorted Fruit Pieces	3	70	0	0	0	0	10	17
Kashi TLC Oatmeal Cookies	30g	130	5	1.5	0	0	70	21
Keebler Animals Shortbread Cookies	31g	160	7	5	0	0	80	22
Keebler Chips Deluxe Chocolate Chip Cookies	16g	80	4.5	2	0	0	50	10
Keebler Chips Deluxe Flavored Coconut Cookies	15g	80	4.5	2	1.5	0	40	9
Keebler Chocolate Lovers Chips Deluxe Chocolate Chip Cookies	16g	80	4.5	2	0	0	65	10
Keebler E.L. Fudge Butter Sandwich Cookies	35g	180	9	3.5	0	5	95	24
Keebler Fudge Shoppe Deluxe Grahams Graham Cookies	27g	140	7	4.5	0	0	70	18
Keebler Fudge Shoppe Flavored Chocolate Cookies	30g	170	10	5	0	0	100	16
Keebler Fudge Shoppe Fudge Sticks Sugar Wafers	29g	150	8	5	0	0	30	20
Keebler Fudge Shoppe Fudge Stripes Shortbread Cookies	31g	150	7	4.5	0	0	110	21
Keebler Fudge Shoppe Right Bites Graham Cookies	20g	100	3.5	2.5	0	0	70	15
Keebler Fudge Shoppe Grasshopper Flavored Mint Cookies	29g	150	7	4.5	0	0	70	20
Keebler Oatmeal Cookies	28g	130	6	2	0	0	100	19
Keebler Pecan Sandies Shortbread Butter Cookies	30g	160	10	3	0	5	105	18
Keebler Rainbow Chips Deluxe Cookies	16g	80	4	1.5	0	0	55	10
Keebler Right Bites Chips Deluxe Chocolate Chip Snack Cookies	21g	100	3	1	0	0	95	17
Keebler Right Bites Fudge Shoppe Shortbread Cookies	21g	100	3.5	2.5	0	0	70	16
Keebler Sandies Shortbread Butter Cookies	30g	160	10	3.5	0	5	90	18
Keebler Simply Sandies Shortbread Butter Cookies	16g	80	4.5	2	2	5	65	10
Keebler Soft Batch Chocolate Chip Cookies	16g	80	3.5	1.5	0	0	55	11
Keebler Vanilla Wafer Golden Cookies	30g	140	6	2	0	0	120	21
Keebler Vienna Fingers Sandwich Cookies	31g	150	6	2	0	0	95	23
Kit Kat Milk Chocolate Wafers	38g	200	12	7	0	10	40	22
Kozy Shack By Request Tapioca Pudding	113g	90	3	2	0	10	130	11
Kozy Shack Old Fashioned Tapioca Pudding	113g	130	3	2	0	15	140	23
Kozy Shack Original Rice Pudding	113g	130	3	2	0	20	135	22
Kozy Shack Real Chocolate Pudding	113g	140	3	2	0	15	140	24
Kozy Shack Rice Pudding	113g	90	3	2	0	15	115	14
Kraft Caramel Pieces	41g	160	3.5	2	0	5	130	31

Packaged Desserts

Packaged Desserts	Serving	Calories	Total fat (gm)	Saturated fat (gm)	Trans fats (gm)	Cholesterol (mg)	Sodium (mg)	Carbs (gm)
Kraft Handi Snacks Oreo Flavored Chocolate Snack Cookies	28g	140	6	1	0	0	120	20
Kraft Jet Puffed White Marshmallows	30g	100	0	0	0	0	25	24
Lifesavers Mint Candy	16g	60	0	0	0	0	0	16
Lindt Lindor Assorted Chocolate Truffles	42g	200	11	7	0	5	30	27
Little Debbie Chocolate Chip Snack Cakes	68g	300	14	8	0	5	210	42
Little Debbie Chocolate Cupcakes	45g	190	9	4.5	0	5	150	26
Little Debbie Chocolate Fudge Brownies	61g	290	13	3.5	0	10	150	40
Little Debbie Chocolate Swiss Rolls	61g	270	12	6	0	15	150	38
Little Debbie Cosmic Brownies	62g	280	11	3.5	0	10	160	42
Little Debbie Devil Squares Devil's Food Snack Cakes	62g	270	12	6	0	0	170	38
Little Debbie Figaroos Snack Cookies	43g	160	3	1	0	0	110	31
Little Debbie Fudge Snack Cakes	43g	190	9	4.5	0	5	125	26
Little Debbie Fudge Snack Cookies	67g	300	11	4	0	5	160	47
Little Debbie Nutty Bar Snack Cookies	60g	320	20	8	0	0	125	33
Little Debbie Oatmeal Snack Cookies	75g	330	12	4	0	0	330	53
Little Debbie Shortcakes	61g	240	9	3	0	15	170	39
Little Debbie Star Crunch Snack Cookies	31g	150	6	3.5	0	0	65	22
Little Debbie Vanilla Fancy Cakes	68g	310	15	8	0	0	160	43
Little Debbie Vanilla Zebra Snack Cakes	74g	320	14	8	0	0	150	48
Little Debbie Yellow Cream Cakes	62g	270	12	4.5	0	15	140	40
Little Debbie Graham Snack Cookies	42g	190	7	4	0	0	190	30
M & M's Chocolate Peanut Candies	36g	220	18	13	0	5	20	15
M & M's Milk Chocolate Candies	42g	220	11	4.5	0	5	20	26
Milky Way Milk Chocolate Caramel Nougat Bars	48g	240	10	6	0	5	30	34
Murray Flavored Ginger Snap Cookies	30g	140	5	1.5	0	0	160	22
Murray Sugar Free Chocolate Chip Cookies	32g	160	9	3.5	0	5	130	20
Murray Sugar Free Flavored Vanilla Sugar Wafers	28g	130	8	2.5	0	0	20	19
Murray Sugar Free Shortbread Cookies	30g	130	5	1.5	0	0	140	21
Murray Sugar Free Wafer Cookies	31g	150	10	7	0	0	20	19
Nabisco Barnum's Animal Crackers	31g	140	4	1	0	0	150	24
Nabisco Candy Blasts Chips Ahoy Chocolate Chip Cookies	17g	90	4.5	2	0	0	50	11
Nabisco Chips Ahoy 100 Calorie Packs	23g	100	3	0.5	0	0	140	18
Nabisco Chips Ahoy Chocolate Chip Cookies	27g	120	5	3	0	0	120	18
Nabisco Chips Ahoy Oatmeal Cookies	27g	120	5	2	0	0	150	17
Nabisco Famous Flavored Chocolate Cookies	32g	140	4.5	1.5	0	5	220	24

Packaged Desserts

	Serving	Calories	Total fat (gm)	Saturated fat (gm)	Trans fats (gm)	Cholesterol (mg)	Sodium (mg)	Carbs (gm)
Nabisco Flavored Ginger Snap Cookies	28g	120	2.5	0.5	0	0	190	23
Nabisco Lorna Doone Shortbread Cookie 100 Calorie Packs	21g	100	3	1.5	0	0	120	16
Nabisco Lorna Doone Shortbread Cookies	29g	140	7	2	0	0	150	20
Nabisco Mallomars Cookies	27g	120	5	3	0	0	40	18
Nabisco Mini Chips Ahoy Chocolate Chip Cookies	31g	150	7	2.5	0	0	105	21
Nabisco Mini Oreo Flavored Chocolate Sandwich Cookies	29g	130	6	2	0	0	160	21
Nabisco Mini Teddy Grahams Snack Cookies	30g	130	4	1	0	0	150	22
Nabisco Newton Cookies	29g	100	1.5	0	0	0	110	21
Nabisco Nilla Snack Cakes	50g	220	10	2	0	5	135	32
Nabisco Nilla Wafer Cookies	29g	110	2	0	0	0	110	24
Nabisco Nutter Butter Bites	30g	140	6	1.5	0	0	115	21
Nabisco Nutter Butter Cookies	32g	160	9	2.5	0	0	90	19
Nabisco Nutter Butter Snack Cookies	53g	250	10	2.5	0	0	210	37
Nabisco Oreo Cakesters Chocolate Snack Cakes	57g	250	12	3	0	5	260	36
Nabisco Oreo Chocolate Snack 100 Calorie Packs	24g	100	4.5	1	0	0	115	15
Nabisco Oreo Cookies	57g	270	11	3.5	0	0	310	41
Nabisco Oreo Double Stuf Cookies	30g	140	6	1.5	0	0	160	21
Nabisco Oreo Fudgees Cookies	31g	140	6	3	0	0	140	22
Nabisco Oreo Thin Wafer 100 Calorie Packs	23g	100	2	0	0	0	160	19
Nabisco Pinwheel Cookies	29g	120	5	2.5	0	0	45	20
Nabisco Products Assorted Snack Cookies	40g	190	9	3	0.5	0	140	27
Nabisco Snackwells Devil's Food Cookies	16g	50	0	0	0	0	25	12
Nabisco Snackwells Sandwich Cookies	25g	110	3	1	0	0	90	20
Nabisco Snackwells Snack Cookies	48g	210	5	1.5	0	0	200	38
Nabisco Teddy Grahams Snack Cookies	30g	130	4.5	1	0	0	160	22
Nabisco Go Paks Mini Oreo Flavored Chocolate Sandwich Cookies	29g	130	6	2	0	0	160	21
Nabisco Golden Oreo Sandwich Cookies	35g	170	7	2	0	0	135	25
Nabsico Mini Nilla Wafer Cookies	30g	140	6	1.5	0	5	115	21
Nestle Butterfinger	37g	170	7	3.5	0	5	85	27
Nestle Crunch Bars	44g	220	11	7	0	5	60	30
Nonni's Biscotti Almond Cookies	24g	110	4.5	2	0	20	70	16
Nonni's Biscotti Cookies	20g	90	3	1	0	20	65	14
Pepperidge Farm Bordeaux Butter Cookies	1 item	32	1	1	0	2	24	5
Pepperidge Farm Brussels Sandwich Cookies	30g	150	7	4	0	5	65	20

Packaged Desserts

Packaged Desserts	Serving	Calories	Total fat (gm)	Saturated fat (gm)	Trans fats (gm)	Cholesterol (mg)	Sodium (mg)	Carbs (gm)
Pepperidge Farm Chessmen Butter Cookies	26g	120	5	3	0	20	80	18
Pepperidge Farm Chocolate Chip Cookies	31g	150	7	3	0	5	70	21
Pepperidge Farm Distinctive Assorted Cookies	25g	130	7	3	0	5	70	16
Pepperidge Farm Milano Cookies	25g	130	7	5	0	5	65	16
Pepperidge Farm Oatmeal Cookies	31g	130	4.5	1.5	0	5	90	23
Pepperidge Farm Pirouette Cookies	25g	120	5	2	0	5	40	19
Peter Paul Almond Joy Bars	45g	220	13	8	0	0	70	26
Peter Paul Mounds Bars	49g	230	13	10	0	0	55	29
Red Vines Red Licorice	40g	140	0	0	0	0	20	34
Reese's Milk Chocolate Peanut Butter Cups	79g	400	24	9	0	5	280	44
Reese's Whipps Milk Chocolate Peanut Butter Nougats	53g	230	9	7	0	0	130	36
Rolo Milk Chocolate Caramels	42g	200	9	6	0	5	70	29
Skittles Fruit Chews	62g	250	2.5	2.5	0	0	10	56
Snickers Chocolate Almond Bars	50g	230	11	4	0	5	115	32
Snickers Chocolate Caramel Peanut Bars	36g	170	9	3.5	0	5	90	22
Starburst Fruit Chews	59g	240	5	4.5	0	0	0	48
T. Marzetti Caramel Apple Dip	38g	140	6	3	0	5	75	22
Tastykake Kandy Kakes	38g	180	10	5	0	10	80	20
Tastykake Krimpets Butterscotch Sponge Cakes	57g	220	6	2.5	0	50	160	39
Three Musketeers Milk Chocolate Nougat Bars	45g	190	6	4	0	5	85	34
Twix Milk Chocolate Caramel Bars	16g	80	4	3	0	0	30	10
Twizzlers Pull N' Peel Cherry Licorice	33g	100	0	0	0	0	85	25
Twizzlers Strawberry Licorice Twists	45g	150	1	0	0	0	115	35
Voortman Sugar Wafers	30g	140	7	1.5	0	0	25	20
Weight Watcher's Chocolate Chip Cookies	25g	90	2.5	1	0	5	150	18
Weight Watcher's Chocolate Snack Cakes	27g	90	3	0.5	0	5	125	17
Weight Watcher's Lemon Finger Cakes	27g	90	3	0	0	5	90	18
Werther's Original Butter & Cream Hard Candies	16g	70	1.5	1	0	5	45	14
York Dark Chocolate Peppermint Patties	39g	140	2.5	1.5	0	0	10	31
York Peppermint Patties	41g	140	3	1.5	0	0	10	32

Grocery Food Factoid:

$756,100,100.00—This is the annual grocery store sales amount for Coke Classic. Coke is the top-selling grocery food out of 400,000 different foods.

Packaged Dinners

	Serving	Calories	Total fat (gm)	Saturated fat (gm)	Trans fats (gm)	Cholesterol (mg)	Sodium (mg)	Carbs (gm)
Betty Crocker Butter & Herb Instant Mashed Potato Mix	25g	90	0.5	0	0	0	390	19
Betty Crocker Cheese Au Gratin Instant Potato Mix	29g	100	0.5	0	0	0	610	23
Betty Crocker Cheese Julienne Instant Potato Mix	25g	80	0	0	0	0	620	20
Betty Crocker Cheesy Scalloped Instant Potato Mix	28g	90	0	0	0	0	650	21
Betty Crocker Chicken Helper Chicken Fried Rice Dinner Mix	30g	100	0.5	0	0	0	490	22
Betty Crocker Chicken Helper Fettuccine Alfredo Dinner Mix	38g	130	1	0	0	0	690	27
Betty Crocker Creamy Au Gratin Instant Potato Mix	28g	90	0.5	0	0	0	580	21
Betty Crocker Creamy Scalloped Instant Potato Mix	28g	90	0	0	0	0	620	22
Betty Crocker Hamburger Helper Bacon Cheeseburger Dinner Mix	34g	120	1	0.5	0	0	760	25
Betty Crocker Hamburger Helper Beef Pasta Dinner Mix	30g	100	0.5	0	0	0	690	21
Betty Crocker Hamburger Helper Cheddar Cheese Melt Dinner Mix	35g	120	1	0	0	0	680	26
Betty Crocker Hamburger Helper Cheese & Hashbrown Dinner Mix	46g	170	1.5	0.5	0	0	870	36
Betty Crocker Hamburger Helper Cheeseburger Macaroni Dinner Mix	32g	110	0.5	0	0	0	800	23
Betty Crocker Hamburger Helper Cheesy Enchilada Dinner Mix	40g	140	1.5	0	0	0	610	30
Betty Crocker Hamburger Helper Cheesy Italian Shell Dinner Mix	33g	110	0.5	0	0	0	770	24
Betty Crocker Hamburger Helper Chili Macaroni Dinner Mix	36g	130	1	0	0	0	640	26
Betty Crocker Hamburger Helper Crunchy Taco Dinner Mix	41g	160	3	0.5	0	0	790	30
Betty Crocker Hamburger Helper Double Cheeseburger Macaroni Dinner Mix	33g	120	1	0	0	0	630	25
Betty Crocker Hamburger Helper Four Cheese Lasagna Dinner Mix	30g	100	1	0	0	0	710	21
Betty Crocker Hamburger Helper Lasagna Dinner Mix	35g	120	0.5	0	0	0	800	26
Betty Crocker Hamburger Helper Philly Cheese Steak Dinner Mix	36g	130	2	1	0	0	670	25
Betty Crocker Hamburger Helper Salisbury Dinner Mix	34g	120	0.5	0	0	0	760	24
Betty Crocker Hamburger Helper Stroganoff Dinner Mix	31g	100	0.5	0	0	0	660	21
Betty Crocker Hamburger Helper 3 Cheese Dinner Mix	34g	120	1	0	0	0	680	24

Packaged Dinners

Packaged Dinners	Serving	Calories	Total fat (gm)	Saturated fat (gm)	Trans fats (gm)	Cholesterol (mg)	Sodium (mg)	Carbs (gm)
Betty Crocker Potato Buds Instant Mashed Potato Mix	23g	80	0	0	0	0	20	18
Betty Crocker Suddenly Salad Classic Salad Mix	53g	180	1	0	0	0	850	38
Betty Crocker Suddenly Salad Ranch with Bacon Salad Mix	47g	170	1.5	0	0	0	370	34
Betty Crocker Three Cheese Scalloped Instant Potato Mix	28g	100	0.5	0	0	0	610	22
Betty Crocker Tuna Helper Creamy Broccoli Dinner Mix	42g	150	1	0	0	0	700	30
Bush's Best Beef Chili with Beans	246g	250	10	4	0	15	810	26
Campbell's Alphabet Vegetable Condensed Soup	120ml	100	0.5	0.5	0	5	890	20
Campbell's Batman Shaped Pasta with Chicken & Chicken Broth Condensed Soup	120ml	70	2	0.5	0	5	580	11
Campbell's Bean Bacon Condensed Soup	120ml	170	4	1.5	0	5	860	25
Campbell's Beef Condensed Broth	120ml	15	0	0	0	0	860	1
Campbell's Beef Condensed Consomme	120ml	20	0	0	0	0	810	1
Campbell's Beef Vegetable & Barley Condensed Soup	120ml	90	1.5	1	0	10	890	15
Campbell's Broccoli & Cheese Condensed Soup	125ml	100	4.5	2	0	5	820	12
Campbell's Cheddar Cheese Condensed Soup	120ml	100	5	2	0	5	890	11
Campbell's Chicken & Stars Condensed Soup	124ml	70	2	0.5	0	5	480	11
Campbell's Chicken Condensed Broth	124ml	20	1	0	0	5	770	1
Campbell's Chicken Noodle Condensed Soup	125ml	60	2	0.5	0	15	890	8
Campbell's Chicken Noodle Soup	240ml	70	2	0.5	0	15	870	10
Campbell's Chicken with Rice Condensed Soup	120ml	70	1.5	0.5	0	5	820	13
Campbell's Chicken Gumbo Condensed Soup	125ml	60	1	0.5	0	5	870	10
Campbell's Chunky Baked Potato with Cheddar & Bacon Bits Soup	240ml	160	6	1	0	5	870	23
Campbell's Chunky Bean & Ham Soup	240ml	180	2	0.5	0	10	780	30
Campbell's Chunky Beef Barley Soup	240ml	170	2.5	1	0	10	890	26
Campbell's Chunky Beef Country Vegetable Soup	240ml	150	2.5	1	0	15	890	21
Campbell's Chunky Chicken & Dumpling Soup	240ml	190	9	2	0	25	890	18
Campbell's Chunky Chicken Broccoli Cheese & Potato Soup	240ml	200	11	4	0	15	910	14
Campbell's Chunky Chili Beef Chili with Beans	240ml	230	8	3.5	0.5	30	870	25

Packaged Dinners

	Serving	Calories	Total fat (gm)	Saturated fat (gm)	Trans fats (gm)	Cholesterol (mg)	Sodium (mg)	Carbs (gm)
Campbell's Chunky Classic Chicken Noodle Soup	240ml	110	2	1	0	25	840	14
Campbell's Chunky Fajita Chicken with Rice & Beans Soup	240ml	140	1.5	0.5	0	15	850	23
Campbell's Chunky Fully Loaded Beef Stew	240ml	160	4	2	0	20	810	20
Campbell's Chunky Fully Loaded Rigatoni & Meatball Soup	240ml	220	8	4	0.5	20	800	24
Campbell's Chunky Fully Loaded Turkey Pot Pie Soup	240ml	200	8	1.5	0	35	800	21
Campbell's Chunky Healthy Request Chicken Corn Chowder	240ml	150	3	1	0	10	480	23
Campbell's Chunky Healthy Request Chicken Noodle Soup	240ml	120	2.5	0.5	0	20	480	15
Campbell's Chunky Healthy Request New England Clam Chowder	240ml	120	2	0.5	0	10	480	20
Campbell's Chunky Healthy Request Vegetable Beef Soup	245ml	120	2	1	0	10	480	19
Campbell's Chunky Healthy Request Grilled Chicken & Sausage Gumbo	245ml	140	2.5	1	0	15	480	21
Campbell's Chunky New England Clam Chowder	240ml	180	8	0.5	0	10	870	20
Campbell's Chunky Pot Roast Soup	240ml	120	1.5	1	0	15	880	18
Campbell's Chunky Savory Chicken with Rice Soup	240ml	110	2	0.5	0	10	810	18
Campbell's Chunky Sirloin Burger & Vegetable Soup	240ml	180	7	3	0	15	900	20
Campbell's Chunky Sirloin Burger with Country Vegetables Soup	240ml	160	4	2	0	15	870	18
Campbell's Chunky Split Pea & Ham Soup	240ml	180	2.5	1	0	10	780	27
Campbell's Chunky Steak & Potato Soup	240ml	130	2	0.5	0	15	920	18
Campbell's Chunky Vegetable Beef Soup	240ml	130	2.5	1	0	15	890	18
Campbell's Chunky Vegetable Soup	240ml	110	1	0.5	0	0	770	22
Campbell's Chunky Grilled Chicken Sausage Gumbo	240ml	140	2.5	1	0	15	850	21
Campbell's Chunky Grilled Sirloin Steak Hearty Vegetable Soup	245ml	130	2	1	0	10	890	19
Campbell's Cream of Broccoli Condensed Soup	120ml	90	3.5	1	0	5	750	12
Campbell's Cream of Celery Condensed Soup	120ml	60	3	1	0	5	580	8
Campbell's Cream of Chicken Condensed Soup	125ml	120	8	2.5	0	10	870	10
Campbell's Cream of Mushroom Condensed Soup	120ml	110	8	1	0	5	650	8
Campbell's Cream of Mushroom with Roasted Garlic Condensed Soup	120ml	70	2.5	1	0	5	710	9

Packaged Dinners

	Serving	Calories	Total fat (gm)	Saturated fat (gm)	Trans fats (gm)	Cholesterol (mg)	Sodium (mg)	Carbs (gm)
Campbell's Cream of Potato Condensed Soup	120ml	90	2	1	0	5	800	15
Campbell's Creamy Tomato Soup	240ml	160	5	1	0	5	750	25
Campbell's Disney Princess Shaped Pasta with Chicken & Chicken Broth Condensed Soup	120ml	70	2	0.5	0	5	580	11
Campbell's Dora The Explorer Nick Jr. Shaped Pasta with Chicken & Chicken Broth Condensed Soup	120ml	70	2	0.5	0	5	580	11
Campbell's Double Noodle Condensed Soup	120ml	100	1.5	0.5	0	10	620	17
Campbell's French Onion Condensed Soup	120ml	45	1.5	1	0	5	900	6
Campbell's Healthy Request Chicken & Rice Condensed Soup	120ml	70	1.5	0.5	0	5	480	13
Campbell's Healthy Request Chicken Noodle Condensed Soup	125ml	60	2	0.5	0	10	480	8
Campbell's Healthy Request Cream of Chicken Condensed Soup	120ml	80	2.5	1	0	5	460	12
Campbell's Healthy Request Cream of Mushroom Condensed Soup	120ml	70	2	0.5	0	5	470	10
Campbell's Healthy Request Tomato Condensed Soup	120ml	90	1.5	0.5	0	0	470	17
Campbell's Homestyle Chicken Noodle Condensed Soup	122g	70	2	1	0	10	940	8
Campbell's Homestyle Chicken Noodle Soup	240ml	70	2	0.5	0	15	890	10
Campbell's Minestrone Condensed Soup	120ml	90	1	0.5	0	5	960	17
Campbell's New England Clam Chowder Condensed Soup	122g	90	2.5	0.5	0	5	880	13
Campbell's Select Harvest Chicken & Egg Noodle Soup	240ml	110	1.5	0.5	0	15	990	14
Campbell's Select Harvest Harvest Tomato with Basil Soup	247ml	100	0	0	0	0	480	22
Campbell's Select Harvest Healthy Request Chicken Tortilla Soup	240ml	130	2	1	0	15	480	20
Campbell's Select Harvest Healthy Request Chicken with Egg Noodles Soup	240ml	90	2	0.5	0	20	480	12
Campbell's Select Harvest Healthy Request Italian Wedding Soup	240ml	110	2.5	1	0	10	480	16
Campbell's Select Harvest Healthy Request Savory Chicken & Long Grain Rice Soup	240ml	120	2	0.5	0	15	480	19
Campbell's Select Harvest Italian Wedding Soup	240ml	160	7	3	0	15	480	16
Campbell's Select Harvest Light Italian Vegetable Soup	240ml	50	0	0	0	0	480	13
Campbell's Select Harvest Light Maryland Crab Soup	240ml	80	0.5	0	0	5	480	16

Packaged Dinners	Serving	Calories	Total fat (gm)	Saturated fat (gm)	Trans fats (gm)	Cholesterol (mg)	Sodium (mg)	Carbs (gm)
Campbell's Select Harvest Light Savory Chicken with Vegetables Soup	240ml	80	1	0.5	0	10	480	15
Campbell's Select Harvest Light Southwest Vegetable Soup	240ml	50	0	0	0	0	480	13
Campbell's Select Harvest Light Vegetable & Pasta Soup	240ml	60	0.5	0	0	5	480	13
Campbell's Select Harvest Light Vegetable Beef Barley Soup	240ml	80	1.5	0.5	0	5	480	14
Campbell's Select Harvest New England Clam Chowder	240ml	170	10	2	0	10	480	15
Campbell's Soup At Hand Chicken & Stars Soup	315ml	70	1.5	0.5	0	5	960	11
Campbell's Soup At Hand Chicken with Mini Noodles Soup	305ml	80	2	1	0	10	980	11
Campbell's Soup At Hand Classic Tomato Soup	305ml	120	0	0	0	0	890	27
Campbell's SpaghettiO's Meatball SpaghettiO's	252g	240	8	3.5	0.5	15	660	32
Campbell's SpaghettiO's Original Cheese & Tomato Sauce	252g	180	1	0	0	5	630	37
Campbell's SpaghettiO's with Meatball & Tomato Sauce	252g	240	8	3.5	0.5	15	660	32
Campbell's Split Pea, Ham & Bacon Condensed Soup	120ml	180	3.5	2	0	5	850	27
Campbell's Tomato Bisque Condensed Soup	120ml	130	3.5	1.5	0	5	880	23
Campbell's Tomato Condensed Soup	120ml	90	0	0	0	0	530	20
Campbell's Tomato Soup	240ml	110	0.5	0	0	0	790	24
Campbell's V8 Southwestern Corn Soup	240ml	150	3	0.5	0	0	620	26
Campbell's V8 Tomato Herb Soup	240ml	90	0	0	0	0	750	19
Campbell's V8 Garden Broccoli Soup	240ml	80	1.5	1	0	5	590	15
Campbell's V8 Golden Butternut Squash Soup	240ml	140	2	1	0	5	750	28
Campbell's Vegetable Beef Condensed Soup	120ml	90	1	0.5	0	5	890	15
Campbell's Vegetarian Vegetable Condensed Soup	120ml	90	0.5	0	0	0	790	18
Campbell's Golden Mushroom Condensed Soup	120ml	80	3.5	1	0	5	890	10
Chef Boyardee ABC & 123 Meatball Pasta with Meatball & Tomato Sauce	247g	260	10	4	0	20	700	32
Chef Boyardee Beef Ravioli Entrée	213g	190	5	2.5	0	10	920	29
Chef Boyardee Beef Ravioli with Tomato & Meat Sauce	252g	250	9	3.5	0	15	950	35
Chef Boyardee Beefaroni Beef & Macaroni Entrée	213g	210	8	3.5	0	15	700	27

Packaged Dinners	Serving	Calories	Total fat (gm)	Saturated fat (gm)	Trans fats (gm)	Cholesterol (mg)	Sodium (mg)	Carbs (gm)
Chef Boyardee Cheese Macaroni & Cheese Entrée	213g	190	8	5	0	15	660	23
Chef Boyardee Macaroni & Cheese	248g	240	10	5	0	15	750	28
Chef Boyardee Meat Spaghetti & Meatball Entrée	213g	200	8	3.5	0	15	820	23
Chef Boyardee Meatball Spaghetti & Meatball Tomato Sauce	255g	270	12	5	0.5	25	980	28
Chef Boyardee Mini Bites Meatball Beef Ravioli with Meatballs & Tomato Sauce	256g	280	12	5	0	25	700	33
Chef Boyardee Mini Bites Meatball Pasta with Meatballs & Tomato Sauce	254g	250	10	4	0	20	690	29
Chef Boyardee Mini Bites Meatball Spaghetti with Meatballs & Tomato Sauce	251g	240	10	4	0	15	750	28
Chef Boyardee Overstuffed Beef Ravioli with Tomato & Meat Sauce	260g	270	6	3	0	20	950	44
College Inn Chicken Ready To Serve Broth	236ml	5	0	0	0	0	450	0
General Mills Romano's Macaroni Grill Creamy Basil Parmesan Chicken Pasta Dinner Mix	43g	150	3.5	1	0	5	830	24
Healthy Choice Chicken & Rice Soup	240g	110	1.5	0	0	10	480	17
Healthy Choice Chicken Noodle Soup	246g	90	2	0.5	0	15	480	12
Healthy Choice Fresh Mixers Rotini & Zesty Marinara Entrée	197g	300	3.5	1	0	0	600	56
Healthy Choice Fresh Mixers Ziti Entrée	197g	340	6	2	0	0	600	56
Hormel Beef Chili No Beans	236g	220	9	4	0	40	970	18
Hormel Beef Chili with Beans	247g	260	7	3	0	30	1160	32
Hormel Compleats Alfredo Chicken & Pasta Entrée	283g	360	20	6	2	45	1300	28
Hormel Compleats Beef & Potato Entrée	283g	230	3	1.5	0	50	1230	27
Hormel Compleats Chicken & Rice Entrée	283g	280	11	3.5	0	40	1170	34
Hormel Compleats Chicken & Dumpling Entrée	283g	260	8	2	0	50	1140	34
Hormel Compleats Chicken & Mashed Potato Entrée	283g	200	3	1	0	30	1100	24
Hormel Compleats Chicken & Noodle Entrée	283g	240	8	4	0	60	1400	27
Hormel Dinty Moore Beef Stew Entrée Can	236g	210	10	4	0	30	970	19
Hormel Hot Beef Chili with Beans	247g	260	7	3	0	30	1190	33
Hormel Mary Kitchen Corned Beef Hash Entrée	236g	390	24	11	1	80	1000	22
Hormel Mary Kitchen Roast Beef Hash Entrée	236g	390	24	10	1	70	790	22
Hormel Turkey Chili with Beans	247g	210	3	1	0	45	1250	28
Hungry Jack Russet Instant Mashed Potato Mix	22g	80	0	0	0	0	20	19
Hunt's Manwich Sloppy Joe Sauce	64g	40	0	0	0	0	410	9

Packaged Dinners	Serving	Calories	Total fat (gm)	Saturated fat (gm)	Trans fats (gm)	Cholesterol (mg)	Sodium (mg)	Carbs (gm)
Hunt's Manwich Zesty Sloppy Joe Sauce	63g	70	0	0	0	0	800	15
Idahoan Baby Reds Creamy Butter Instant Mashed Potato Mix	29g	110	3	1	0	0	400	21
Idahoan Buttery Homestyle Instant Mashed Potato Mix	28g	110	3	1	0	0	450	20
Idahoan Four Cheese Instant Mashed Potato Mix	28g	110	2.5	1	0	0	590	20
Idahoan Loaded Baked Butter Sour Cream, Cheese, Bacon & Chives Instant Mashed Potato Mix	28g	110	2.5	1	0	0	500	20
Idahoan Roasted Garlic Instant Mashed Potato Mix	28g	110	3	1	0	0	590	20
Kitchen Basics Beef Soup Stock	237ml	20	0	0	0	0	480	1
Kitchen Basics Chicken Soup Stock	240ml	20	0	0	0	0	480	1
Knorr Lipton Asian Sides Teriyaki Side Dish Mix	66g	240	2	0	0	0	790	48
Knorr Lipton Italian Sides Creamy Garlic Side Dish Mix	69g	260	4.5	2.5	0	10	660	47
Knorr Lipton Pasta Sides Alfredo Side Dish Mix	62g	240	4.5	2.5	0	10	810	40
Knorr Lipton Pasta Sides Butter & Herb Side Dish Mix	62g	230	3.5	1.5	0	5	660	44
Knorr Lipton Pasta Sides Butter Side Dish Mix	63g	240	4	2	0	10	770	43
Knorr Lipton Pasta Sides Cheddar Broccoli Side Dish Mix	68g	250	2.5	1	0	5	780	48
Knorr Lipton Pasta Sides Chicken Broccoli Side Dish Mix	59g	210	2	0	0	5	780	42
Knorr Lipton Pasta Sides Chicken Side Dish Mix	59g	210	2	1	0	5	850	41
Knorr Lipton Pasta Sides Parmesan Side Dish Mix	60g	220	4.5	2.5	0	10	680	37
Knorr Lipton Pasta Sides Stroganoff Side Dish Mix	56g	210	2	1	0	5	760	39
Kraft Deluxe Cheese Elbow Macaroni & Cheese Mix	98g	290	4.5	2	0	15	850	50
Kraft Deluxe Four Cheese Elbow Macaroni & Cheese Mix	98g	320	10	3.5	0	15	850	47
Kraft Deluxe Original Elbow Macaroni & Cheese Mix	98g	320	10	3	0	15	930	45
Kraft Deluxe Sharp Cheddar Cheese Elbow Macaroni & Cheese Mix	98g	320	9	3	0	15	840	47
Kraft Easy Mac Extreme Cheese Elbow Macaroni & Cheese Mix	61g	230	4	2.5	0	5	520	42
Kraft Easy Mac Original Elbow Macaroni & Cheese Mix	61g	230	4	2.5	0	5	550	42
Kraft Easy Mac Original Macaroni & Cheese Mix	58g	220	4	2.5	0	5	700	39

Packaged Dinners

	Serving	Calories	Total fat (gm)	Saturated fat (gm)	Trans fats (gm)	Cholesterol (mg)	Sodium (mg)	Carbs (gm)
Kraft Easy Mac Original Tube Macaroni & Cheese Mix	58g	220	4	2.5	0	5	700	39
Kraft Easy Mac Triple Cheese Macaroni & Cheese Mix	58g	220	4.5	2.5	0	5	660	39
Kraft Original Elbow Macaroni & Cheese Mix	70g	260	3.5	2	0	15	580	48
Kraft Original Tube Macaroni & Cheese Mix	70g	260	3.5	2	0	15	580	48
Kraft Pasta Salad Ranch with Bacon Pasta Side Dish	47g	160	0.5	0	0	0	300	33
Kraft Premium 3 Cheese Shell Macaroni & Cheese Mix	70g	260	2.5	1	0	5	610	50
Kraft Scooby Doo Mystery Shapes Macaroni & Cheese Mix	70g	260	2.5	1.5	0	10	580	49
Kraft Spiderman Macaroni & Cheese Mix	70g	260	2.5	1.5	0	10	580	49
Kraft Spiral Macaroni & Cheese Mix	70g	260	3.5	2	0	15	580	48
Kraft Spongebob Squarepants Macaroni & Cheese Mix	70g	260	2.5	1.5	0	10	580	49
Kraft Stove Top Chicken Stuffing Mix	28g	110	2.5	0	0	0	460	20
Kraft Stove Top Cornbread Stuffing Mix	28g	100	1	0	0	0	500	22
Kraft Stove Top Pork Stuffing Mix	28g	100	1	0	0	0	430	21
Kraft Stove Top Savory Herb Stuffing Mix	28g	110	1	0	0	0	450	21
Kraft Stove Top Turkey Stuffing Mix	28g	110	1	0	0	0	440	21
Kraft Thick N' Creamy Elbow Macaroni & Cheese Mix	70g	250	2	1	0	5	580	50
Kraft Velveeta Broccoli & Cheese Rotini Macaroni & Cheese Mix	126g	400	16	5	0	25	1230	49
Kraft Velveeta Cheese Shell Macaroni & Cheese Mix	112g	330	4.5	2	0	15	990	58
Kraft Velveeta Original Shell Macaroni & Cheese Mix	112g	360	12	4	0	20	940	49
Kraft Whole Grain Elbow Macaroni & Cheese Mix	70g	260	3.5	2	0	15	590	49
La Choy Chicken Chow Mein Dinner Oriental Food Product	250g	100	3	1	0	20	1210	10
Libby's Corned Beef Hash Entrée Can	252g	420	24	11	1	55	1230	33
Near East Parmesan Side Dish Mix	56g	200	2	0.5	0	5	580	39
Near East Roasted Garlic & Olive Oil Side Dish Mix	56g	200	2	0	0	0	570	39
Near East Side Dish Mix	62g	220	1	0	0	0	5	46
Near East Toasted Pine Nut Side Dish Mix	56g	200	2.5	0.5	0	0	510	39
Pacific Natural Foods Chicken Ready To Serve Broth	240ml	15	0	0	0	0	70	1
Pepperidge Farm Herb Stuffing Mix	27g	130	5	3.5	0	10	95	19
Progresso Beef Barley Soup	242g	140	3.5	1.5	0	15	650	18

Packaged Dinners

Packaged Dinners	Serving	Calories	Total fat (gm)	Saturated fat (gm)	Trans fats (gm)	Cholesterol (mg)	Sodium (mg)	Carbs (gm)
Progresso Beef Pot Roast with Vegetables Soup	247g	120	1.5	0.5	0	15	830	20
Progresso Chickarina Soup	237g	120	5	2	0	20	950	12
Progresso Chicken & Sausage Gumbo	249g	130	4	1.5	0	15	900	18
Progresso Chicken & Wild Rice Soup	239g	100	1.5	0.5	0	15	650	15
Progresso Chicken Corn Chowder	255g	200	9	2.5	0	15	790	23
Progresso Chicken Herb Dumpling Soup	234g	100	2.5	1	0	30	790	14
Progresso Chicken Noodle Soup	246g	110	2.5	0.5	0	30	690	14
Progresso Chicken Pot Pie Soup	245g	150	5	1	0	15	890	20
Progresso Chicken Ready To Serve Broth	240g	20	0	0	0	0	850	1
Progresso Chicken Rice Vegetable Soup	238g	100	1	0.5	0	15	870	16
Progresso Cream of Mushroom Soup	230g	130	10	3	0	10	820	9
Progresso French Onion Soup	210g	50	1.5	0.5	0	5	900	9
Progresso Healthy Favorites Chicken & Wild Rice Ready To Serve Soup	247g	90	1.5	0	0	15	470	14
Progresso Healthy Favorites Chicken Noodle Soup	240g	90	1.5	0	0	20	470	12
Progresso Healthy Favorites Chicken Gumbo	248ml	110	1.5	0.5	0	15	450	18
Progresso Healthy Favorites Italian Style Wedding with Meat Ready To Serve Soup	247g	90	2	1	0	10	480	11
Progresso Healthy Favorites Minestrone Soup	252g	120	2	0.5	0	0	470	24
Progresso Healthy Favorites Garden Vegetable Ready To Serve Soup	250g	100	0	0	0	0	450	22
Progresso Hearty Chicken & Rotini Soup	235g	100	2	0.5	0	15	690	13
Progresso Homestyle Chicken Soup	240g	100	2	0	0	10	830	14
Progresso Lentil Soup	242g	150	1.5	0	0	0	500	26
Progresso Light Beef Pot Roast Soup	240g	80	1	0	0	15	690	12
Progresso Light Chicken Noodle Soup	236g	70	1.5	0.5	0	20	680	10
Progresso Light Chicken Vegetable Rotini Soup	236g	70	1.5	0.5	0	15	700	10
Progresso Light Savory Vegetable Barley Soup	243ml	60	0	0	0	0	690	14
Progresso Light Southwest Vegetable Soup	242g	60	0	0	0	0	690	12
Progresso Light Vegetable & Noodle Soup	248g	60	0.5	0	0	5	690	13
Progresso Light Vegetable & Rice Soup	242g	60	0	0	0	0	690	14
Progresso Light Vegetable Soup	238ml	60	0	0	0	0	470	14
Progresso Light Zesty Chicken Soup	236g	80	1	0	0	10	680	10
Progresso Manhattan Clam Chowder	239g	100	2	0	0	10	970	17
Progresso Minestrone Soup	240ml	100	2	0.5	0	0	980	18
Progresso New England Clam Chowder	240g	190	9	2	0	10	980	22

Packaged Dinners

Packaged Dinners	Serving	Calories	Total fat (gm)	Saturated fat (gm)	Trans fats (gm)	Cholesterol (mg)	Sodium (mg)	Carbs (gm)
Progresso Savory Beef Barley Vegetable Soup	245g	130	1	0.5	0	15	970	22
Progresso Split Pea & Ham Soup	243g	140	1	0	0	5	690	24
Progresso Split Green Pea Soup	244ml	160	2	0.5	0	0	840	28
Progresso Vegetable Soup	238g	80	0.5	0	0	0	610	16
Progresso Garden Vegetable Soup	235ml	100	0	0	0	0	900	21
Rice-A-Roni Pasta Roni Fettuccine Alfredo Side Dish Mix	70g	260	6	3	0	5	910	44
Rice-A-Roni Pasta Roni Herb Side Dish Mix	56g	190	2.5	1	0	0	680	38
Rice-A-Roni Pasta Roni Olive Oil & Garlic Side Dish Mix	70g	240	3	1	0	0	880	47
Rice-A-Roni Pasta Roni Parmesan Cheese Side Dish Mix	56g	200	4	2	0	0	740	36
Rice-A-Roni Pasta Roni White Cheddar Side Dish Mix	56g	200	4.5	2	0	5	630	36
Swanson Beef Ready To Serve Broth	198g	15	0	0	0	0	440	1
Swanson Beef Soup Stock	236ml	25	0	0	0	0	500	2
Swanson Chicken Ready To Serve Broth	233g	15	0.5	0	0	5	960	1
Swanson Chicken Soup Stock	236ml	20	0	0	0	0	510	1
Swanson Natural Goodness Chicken Ready To Serve Broth	240ml	15	0	0	0	0	570	1
Swanson Vegetable Broth	198g	15	0	0	0	0	940	3

Grocery Food Factoid:

What do these 7 foods have in common?

Bertolli Oven Bake Meals Frozen Tri Color Four Cheese Ravioli Entrée

Dreyer's/Edy's Dibs Vanilla Bites Frozen Ice Cream

Bertolli Frozen Chicken Florentine and Farfalle Entrée

Edward's Frozen Oreo Cream Pie

Edward's Frozen Chocolate Cream Pie

Boston Market Frozen Meatloaf & Mashed Potato Entrée

Marie Callender's One-Dish Classics Frozen Chicken & Fettucine Entrée

They have the most saturated fat of any foods in this guide.

Pasta & Rice	Serving	Calories	Total fat (gm)	Saturated fat (gm)	Trans fats (gm)	Cholesterol (mg)	Sodium (mg)	Carbs (gm)
arilla Angel Hair Pasta	56g	200	1	0	0	0	0	42
arilla Elbow Macaroni	56g	200	1	0	0	0	0	42
arilla Farfalle Bowtie Pasta	56g	200	1	0	0	0	0	42
arilla Fettuccine Pasta	56g	200	1	0	0	0	0	42
arilla Lasagne Sheets	51g	190	1.5	0	0	15	10	38
arilla Linguine Pasta	56g	200	1	0	0	0	0	42
arilla Macaroni	56g	200	1	0	0	0	0	42
arilla Mezze Penne Pasta	56g	200	1	0	0	0	0	42
arilla Plus Multigrain Angel Hair Pasta	56g	210	2	0	0	0	25	38
arilla Plus Multigrain Elbow Macaroni	56g	210	2	0	0	0	25	38
arilla Plus Multigrain Penne Pasta	56g	210	2	0	0	0	25	38
arilla Plus Multigrain Rotini Pasta	56g	210	2	0	0	0	25	38
arilla Plus Multigrain Spaghetti	56g	210	2	0	0	0	25	38
arilla Rigatoni Pasta	56g	200	1	0	0	0	0	42
arilla Rotini Pasta	56g	200	1	0	0	0	0	42
arilla Spaghetti	56g	200	1	0	0	0	0	42
arilla Whole Grain Penne Pasta	56g	200	1.5	0	0	0	0	41
arilla Whole Grain Rotini Pasta	56g	200	1.5	0	0	0	0	41
arilla Whole Grain Spaghetti	56g	200	1.5	0	0	0	0	41
arilla Ziti Pasta	56g	200	1	0	0	0	0	42
uitoni Fettuccine	83g	240	2.5	1	0	45	20	44
uitoni Chicken & Herb Tortellini	110g	350	10	2.5	0	40	380	52
uitoni Chicken & Proscuitto Tortelloni	109g	330	9	3	0	40	650	46
uitoni Four Cheese Ravioli	105g	340	12	4	0	55	650	42
uitoni Spinach & Cheese Tortellini	106g	320	7	3.5	0	55	510	49
uitoni Three Cheese Tortellini	106g	330	9	3	0	40	460	46
anilla Extra Long Grain White Rice	45g	160	0	0	0	0	0	35
reamette Macaroni	56g	210	1	0	0	0	0	42
reamette Spaghetti	56g	210	1	0	0	0	0	42
reamfields Spaghetti	56g	190	1	0	0	0	10	41
oya Long Grain Spanish Yellow Rice Mix	45g	160	0	0	0	0	820	36
uerrero Yellow Corn Tostada Shells	32g	160	7	2	0	0	240	20
ormel Mexican Beef Tamales	142g	140	7	3	0	15	710	15
ikkoman Oriental Stir-Fry Sauce	15ml	20	0	0	0	0	520	4
norr Lipton Asian Sides Chicken Fried Rice & Sauce Mix	66g	220	1.5	0	0	5	750	47
norr Lipton Fiesta Sides Mexican Rice Mix	68g	240	1	0	0	0	940	52
norr Lipton Fiesta Sides Spanish Rice & Pasta Mix	67g	240	1	0	0	0	830	52

Pasta & Rice	Serving	Calories	Total fat (gm)	Saturated fat (gm)	Trans fats (gm)	Cholesterol (mg)	Sodium (mg)	Carbs (gm)
Knorr Lipton Rice Sides Cheddar, Broccoli, Rice & Sauce Mix	68g	230	1.5	0.5	0	5	860	48
Knorr Lipton Rice Sides Chicken, Broccoli, Rice & Pasta Mix	65g	210	1	0	0	5	830	46
Knorr Lipton Rice Sides Creamy Chicken & White Rice Mix	68g	250	2	0.5	0	0	680	52
La Choy Chow Mein Noodles	28g	130	5	1.5	1.5	0	230	19
Light & Fluffy Egg Noodles	56g	210	2.5	1	0	70	15	40
Lipton Rice Sides Chicken Rice Mix	65g	230	2.5	0.5	0	5	820	47
Mahatma Thai Jasmine Long Grain Rice	45g	160	0	0	0	0	0	36
Minute Regular Whole Grain Brown Rice	43g	150	1.5	0	0	0	10	34
Mueller's Angel Hair Pasta	57g	210	1	0	0	0	0	41
Mueller's Macaroni	56g	210	1	0	0	0	0	41
Mueller's Spaghetti	56g	210	1	0	0	0	0	41
Near East Original Rice Pilaf	56g	190	0.5	0	0	0	780	43
No Yolks Dumpling Noodles	56g	210	0.5	0	0	0	30	41
No Yolks Egg Substitute Noodles	56g	210	0.5	0	0	0	30	41
Old El Paso Assorted Dinner Kit	49g	130	5	2	0	0	760	18
Old El Paso Corn Taco Shells	32g	150	7	3	0	0	135	19
Old El Paso Flour Taco Kit	82g	180	5	1	1	0	1170	32
Old El Paso Refried Beans	124g	90	0	0	0	0	580	17
Old El Paso Refried Beans with No Additives	120g	90	0.5	0	0	0	560	16
Old El Paso Stand N' Stuff Yellow Corn Dinner Kit	60g	160	6	2.5	0	0	900	23
Old El Paso Stand N' Stuff Yellow Corn Taco Shells	27g	130	6	2.5	0	0	115	16
Ortega Corn Taco Kit	28g	160	7	1	0	0	640	22
Ortega Yellow Corn Taco Shells	28g	120	6	1	0	0	170	16
Rice-A-Roni Beef, Long Grain Rice & Vermicelli Mix	70g	230	1	0	0	0	930	51
Rice-A-Roni Chicken, Broccoli, Rice & Vermicelli Mix	56g	180	1	0	0	0	870	40
Rice-A-Roni Chicken, Rice & Vermicelli Mix	70g	230	1	0	0	0	960	50
Rice-A-Roni Creamy Four Cheese Rice Mix	56g	210	4.5	2.5	0	5	660	37
Rice-A-Roni Fried Rice & Vermicelli Mix	70g	230	1	0	0	0	1240	50
Rice-A-Roni Herb Butter, Rice & Pasta Mix	70g	240	1.5	0.5	0	0	960	53
Rice-A-Roni Lower Sodium Chicken & Rice Mix	70g	230	1.5	0	0	0	620	50
Rice-A-Roni Spanish Rice & Vermicelli Mix	56g	180	1	0	0	0	890	40
Ronzoni Healthy Harvest Whole Wheat Penne Pasta	56g	180	2	0	0	0	0	41

Pasta & Rice

	Serving	Calories	Total fat (gm)	Saturated fat (gm)	Trans fats (gm)	Cholesterol (mg)	Sodium (mg)	Carbs (gm)
ꞏnzoni Healthy Harvest Whole Wheat ꞏpaghetti	56g	180	2	0	0	0	0	41
ꞏnzoni Lasagne	56g	210	1	0	0	0	0	42
ꞏnzoni Macaroni	56g	210	1	0	0	0	0	42
ꞏnzoni Spaghetti	56g	210	1	0	0	0	0	42
ꞏsarita Traditional Refried Beans with No ꞏdditives	128g	100	0	0	0	0	510	19
ꞏan Giorgio Macaroni	56g	210	1	0	0	0	0	42
ꞏoy Vay Oriental Teriyaki Marinade & ꞏauce	15 ml	35	1	0	0	0	490	6
ꞏuccess Whole Grain Brown Rice	43g	150	1	0	0	0	0	33
ꞏco Bell Home Originals Corn Dinner Kit	50g	130	4.5	0.5	0	0	530	20
ꞏco Bell Home Originals Corn Taco Shells	32g	150	6	1	0	0	5	22
ꞏco Bell Home Originals Refried Beans	130g	120	1	0	0	0	610	20
ꞏncle Ben's Converted Original Long Grain ꞏhite Rice	49g	170	0	0	0	0	0	38
ꞏncle Ben's Natural Whole Grain Brown ꞏce	47g	170	1.5	0	0	0	0	35
ꞏncle Ben's Original Long Grain Wild Rice ꞏix	57g	200	0	0	0	0	670	44
ꞏncle Ben's Ready Rice Brown Rice Mix	140g	240	3	0	0	0	15	39
ꞏncle Ben's Ready Rice Long Grain Rice ꞏlaf Mix	155g	220	3.5	0.5	0	0	970	42
ꞏncle Ben's Ready Rice Long Grain Wild ꞏce Mix	153g	220	3	0	0	0	900	43
ꞏncle Ben's Ready Rice Original White ꞏce Mix	140g	200	2.5	0	0	0	10	40
ꞏncle Ben's Ready Rice Roasted Chicken ꞏce Mix	151g	220	3.5	0	0	0	1020	41
ꞏncle Ben's Ready Rice Spanish Rice Mix	144g	200	2.5	0	0	0	680	41
ꞏncle Ben's Ready Rice Whole Grain ꞏown & Wild Rice Medley	146g	220	3.5	0	0	0	730	42
ꞏncle Ben's Ready Rice Garden Vegetable ꞏce Mix	145g	200	2.5	0	0	0	830	41
ꞏacky Mac Vegetable Macaroni	56g	200	1	0	0	0	15	41
ꞏatarain's New Orleans Dirty Rice Mix	38g	130	0	0	0	0	620	29
ꞏatarain's New Orleans Jambalaya Rice Mix	38g	130	0	0	0	0	500	29
ꞏatarain's New Orleans Long Grain Rice & ꞏean Mix	66g	220	0.5	0	0	0	1190	47
ꞏatarain's New Orleans Long Grain Yellow ꞏce Mix	57g	190	0	0	0	0	930	43
ꞏatarain's Red Bean Long Grain White Rice ꞏ Bean Mix	57g	190	0	0	0	0	1190	40

Produce	Serving	Calories	Total fat (gm)	Saturated fat (gm)	Trans fats (gm)	Cholesterol (mg.)	Sodium (mg)	Carbs (gm)
Alfalfa, Sprouted	1 cup	9	0	0	0	0	2	1
Almonds	1 cup	826	72	6	0	0	1	2
Amaranth	1 cup	6	0	0	0	0	6	1
Apples	1 item	72	0	0	0	0	1	19
Apricots	1 item	17	0	0	0	0	0	4
Artichokes	1 item	60	0	0	0	0	120	13
Asparagus	1 cup	26	0	0	0	0	3	5
Avocados	1 item	289	26.5	3.5	0	0	14	15
Bamboo Shoots	1 cup	40	0	0	0	0	6	8
Bananas	1 item	105	0	0	0	0	1	27
Barley (Pearled)	1 cup	704	2	0	0	0	18	15
Beans	1 cup	50	1	0	0	0	11	25
Beets	1 cup	58	0	0	0	0	106	13
Black Currants	1 cup	70	0	0	0	0	2	17
Blackberries	1 cup	62	0.5	0	0	0	1	14
Blueberries	½ pint	83	0.5	0	0	0	1	21
Bok Choy	1 cup	9	0	0	0	0	46	2
Boysenberries	1 cup	66	0	0	0	0	1	16
Brazil Nuts	1 cup	918	93	21	0	0	4	17
Broccoli	1 cup	29	0	0	0	0	29	6
Brussel Sprouts	1 cup	37	0	0	0	0	22	8
Butternut Squash	1 cup	82	0	0	0	0	8	24
Cabbage	1 cup	21	0	0	0	0	16	5
Cantaloupe	1 cup	60	0	0	0	0	28	15
Carrots	1 item	25	0	0	0	0	42	6
Cashews	1 cup	720	56	6	0	0	0	8
Cauliflower	1 cup	25	0	0	0	0	30	5
Celery	1 stalk	5	0	0	0	0	32	1
Chard	1 cup	6	0	0	0	0	77	1
Cherries	1cup	74	0	0	0	0	0	23
Chestnuts	1 cup	308	3	1	0	0	4	66
Chinese Cabbage	1 cup	16	0	0	0	0	9	1
Clementines	1 item	35	0	0	0	0	1	5
Coconut	1 cup	283	27	24	0	0	16	12
Collards	1 cup	10	0	0	0	0	7	2
Corn	1 cup	132	2	0	0	0	23	29
Cranberries	1 cup	44	0	0	0	0	2	13
Cress	1 cup	16	0	0	0	0	17	3
Cucumbers	1 item	45	0	0	0	0	6	11
Currants	1 cup	62	0	0	0	0	1	15

Produce

Produce	Serving	Calories	Total fat (gm)	Saturated fat (gm)	Trans fats (gm)	Cholesterol (mg)	Sodium (mg)	Carbs (gm)
Dates	½ cup	251	0	0	0	0	2	75
Dole Classic Salad Mix	85g	15	0	0	0	0	15	4
Dole Coleslaw Mix	85g	25	0	0	0	0	25	5
Dole Complete Caesar Salad Mix	100g	160	13	2.5	0	10	290	7
Dole Fresh Discoveries Butter & Red Leaf Salad Mix	85g	10	0	0	0	0	10	3
Dole Fresh Discoveries Field Green Salad Mix	85g	20	0	0	0	0	15	4
Dole Fresh Discoveries Hearts Delight Salad Mix	85g	15	0	0	0	0	10	3
Dole Fresh Discoveries Hearts of Romaine Salad Mix	85g	15	0	0	0	0	5	3
Dole Fresh Discoveries Italian Salad Mix	85g	15	0	0	0	0	10	3
Dole Fresh Discoveries Leafy Romaine Salad Mix	85g	15	0	0	0	0	15	3
Dole Fresh Discoveries Mediterranean Blend Salad Mix	85g	15	0	0	0	0	20	3
Dole Fresh Discoveries Romaine Salad Mix	85g	15	0	0	0	0	10	4
Dole Fresh Discoveries Salad Mix	85g	20	0	0	0	0	10	4
Dole Fresh Discoveries Single Caesar Salad Kit	100g	90	6	1	0	5	340	8
Dole Fresh Discoveries Spinach Salad Mix	85g	20	0	0	0	0	65	3
Dole Fresh Discoveries Garden Salad Mix	85g	15	0	0	0	0	30	2
Dole Fresh Favorites American Salad Mix	85g	15	0	0	0	0	10	3
Dole Fresh Favorites Greener Selection Salad Mix	85g	15	0	0	0	0	15	4
Dole Fresh Makes Complete Caesar Salad	100g	160	13	2.5	0	10	290	7
Dole Fresh Makes Harvest Salad Kit	100g	160	12	1.5	0	0	105	12
Dole Fresh Makes Southwest Salad Kit	100g	150	11	2.5	0	10	340	10
Dole Salad Very Veggie Mix	85g	20	0	0	0	0	15	4
Dole Shredded Lettuce Mix	85g	15	0	0	0	0	10	3
Earthbound Farm Organic Baby Lettuce Blend	85g	15	0	0	0	0	60	3
Earthbound Farm Organic Baby Spinach Salad Kit	85g	10	0	0	0	0	100	7
Earthbound Farm Organic Lettuce Mix	85g	15	0	0	0	0	70	4
Earthbound Farm Organic Romaine Salad Mix	85g	15	0	0	0	0	50	2
Earthbound Farm Organic Rugula Salad Mix	85g	20	0	0	0	0	25	3
Earthbound Farm Organic Spring Blend Salad Mix	85g	15	0	0	0	0	70	4
Eggplant	1 item	109	1	0	0	0	9	31
Fennel	1 item	73	0	0	0	0	122	17
Figs	1 item	37	1.5	0	0	0	1	10

Produce

Produce	Serving	Calories	Total fat (gm)	Saturated fat (gm)	Trans fats (gm)	Cholesterol (mg)	Sodium (mg)	Carbs (gm)
Flax Seed	30ml	90	7	0	0	0	0	5
French Beans	10	17	0	0	0	0	5	6
Gooseberries	1 cup	66	1	0	0	0	2	15
Grapefruit	1 half	41	0	0	0	0	0	16
Grapes	1 cup	62	0	0	0	0	2	29
Green Peppers	1 item	24	0	0	0	0	24	6
Guava	1 cup	112	2	0	0	0	3	24
Hazelnuts	1 cup	847	82	6	0	0	0	23
Honeydew Melon	1 cup	64	0	0	0	0	32	16
Huckleberries	1 cup	81	0.5	0	0	0	9	20
Jerusalem Artichoke	1 cup	114	0	0	0	0	6	26
Jicama	1 item	250	1	0	0	0	26	58
Kale	1 cup	33	0	0	0	0	29	7
Kiwi Fruit	1 item	46	0	0	0	0	2	11
Kumquats	1 item	13	0	0	0	0	2	3
Leeks	1 item	54	0	0	0	0	18	13
Lemons	1 item	24	0	0	0	0	2	11
Lettuce	1 cup	7	0	0	0	0	4	2
Lima Beans	1 cup	176	1	0	0	0	12	31
Limes	1 item	20	0	0	0	0	1	7
Loganberries	1 cup	80	0	0	0	0	1	19
Macadamia Nuts	1 cup	962	102	16	0	0	7	19
Mangos	1 cup	107	0	0	0	0	3	28
Melons	1 cup	64	0	0	0	0	32	16
Millet	1 cup	756	8	1	0	0	10	146
Mulberries	1 cup	60	1	0	0	0	14	14
Mushrooms	1 cup	21	0	0	0	0	4	2
Nectarines	1 cup	61	0	0	0	0	0	15
Oats	1 cup	606	11	2	0	0	3	103
Okra	1 cup	31	0	0	0	0	8	7
Olives	1 item	4	0	0	0	0	39	0
Onions	1 item	46	0	0	0	0	3	11
Oranges	1 item	62	0	0	0	0	0	18
Papaya	1 cup	55	0	0	0	0	4	30
Parsnips	1 cup	99	0	0	0	0	13	24
Passionfruit	1 cup	228	2	0	0	0	66	55
Peaches	1 item	38	0	0	0	0	0	9
Peanuts	1 cup	862	76	13	0	0	461	24
Pears	1 item	81	0	0	0	0	1	21
Peas	1 cup	117	1	0	0	0	7	21

Produce

Produce	Serving	Calories	Total fat (gm)	Saturated fat (gm)	Trans fats (gm)	Cholesterol (mg)	Sodium (mg)	Carbs (gm)
Pecans	1 cup	753	78	7	0	0	0	15
Peppers	1 item	24	0	0	0	0	24	2
Persimmons	1 item	31	0	0	0	0	0	8
Pine Nuts / Pignolias	1 cup	909	92	7	0	0	3	18
Pineapple	1 cup	74	0	0	0	0	2	20
Pistachios	1 cup	685	55	7	0	0	1	34
Plums	1 item	30	0	0	0	0	0	8
Pomegranates	1 item	105	0	0	0	0	5	26
Potatoes	1 item	161	0	0	0	0	17	37
Pumpkin	1 cup	30	0	0	0	0	1	8
Quinoa	1 cup	635	10	1	0	0	36	117
Radicchio	1 cup	9	0	0	0	0	9	2
Radishes	1 cup	18	0	0	0	0	45	4
Raspberries	1 cup	64	0.8	0	0	0	1	15
Red Currants	1 cup	63	0	0	0	0	1	14
Rhubarb	1 cup	25	0	0	0	0	5	6
Rye	1 cup	566	4	0	0	0	10	118
Shallots	100g	72	0	0	0	0	12	17
Spaghetti Squash	1 cup	42	0	0	0	0	28	7
Spinach	1 cup	6	0	0	0	0	24	4
Spirulina (Seaweed)	100g	45	1	0	0	0	872	24
Squash	1 cup	42	0	0	0	0	28	16
Starfruit / Carambola	1 item	28	0	0	0	0	2	6
Strawberries	1 cup	49	0	0	0	0	2	11
Summer Squash	1 cup	18	0	0	0	0	2	4
Sweet Corn	1 item	77	1	0	0	0	14	19
Sweet Potatoes	1 item	111	0	0	0	0	72	26
Swiss Chard	1 cup	6	0	0	0	0	77	1
Tangerines	1 item	45	0	0	0	0	2	11
Taro	1 cup	116	0	0	0	0	11	28
Tomatoes	1 item	22	0	0	0	0	6	2
Turnips	1 item	34	0	0	0	0	82	8
Walnuts	1 cup	654	65	6	0	0	2	16
Watercress	1 cup	3	0	0	0	0	14	0
Watermelon	1 cup	46	0	0	0	0	2	11
Wheat - Durum	1 cup	650	5	1	0	0	4	137
Wheat - Hard Red	1 cup	627	3	1	0	0	4	137
Wheat - Hard White	1 cup	656	3	1	0	0	4	146
Winter Squash	1 cup	31	1	0	0	0	17	10
Yams	1 cup	177	0	0	0	0	14	42
Yellow Squash	1 item	31	0	0	0	0	12	7
Zucchini	1 item	31	0	0	0	0	12	0

Snacks

	Serving	Calories	Total fat (gm)	Saturated fat (gm)	Trans fats (gm)	Cholesterol (mg)	Sodium (mg)	Carbs (gm)
Baked Cheetos	28g	130	5	1	0	0	240	19
Baked Doritos	28g	120	3.5	0.5	0	0	220	21
Baked Lay's Barbecue Potato Chips	28g	120	3	0.5	0	0	210	22
Baked Lay's Cheddar & Sour Cream Potato Chips	28g	120	3.5	1	0	0	210	21
Baked Lay's Original Potato Chips	28g	120	2	0	0	0	180	23
Baked Lay's Sour Cream & Onion Potato Chips	28g	120	3	0.5	0	0	210	21
Baked Ruffles Cheddar & Sour Cream Chips	28g	120	3	0.5	0	0	220	22
Baked Ruffles Original Potato Chips	28g	120	3	0	0	0	200	21
Tostito's Scoops Tortilla Chips	28g	120	3	0.5	0	0	125	22
Baken-Ets Hot N' Spicy Fried Pork Rinds	14g	80	5	2	0	20	470	0
Baken-Ets Traditional Fried Pork Rinds	14g	80	5	2.5	0	20	310	0
Betty Crocker Batman Fruit Snacks	25g	80	0	0	0	0	30	21
Betty Crocker Fruit By The Foot Roll Fruit Flavored Snacks	21g	80	1	0	0	0	45	17
Betty Crocker Fruit Roll-Ups Fruit Snacks	14g	50	1	0	0	0	55	12
Betty Crocker Fruit Gushers Fruit Snacks	25g	90	1	0	0.5	0	45	20
Betty Crocker Scooby Doo Fruit Snacks	25g	80	0	0	0	0	30	21
Betty Crocker Spiderman Fruit Snacks	25g	80	0	0	0	0	30	21
Blue Diamond Almond Nut Snacks	28g	170	16	1	0	0	85	5
Blue Diamond Smokehouse Almond Nut Snacks	28g	170	16	1	0	0	150	5
Blue Diamond Wasabi & Soy Sauce Almond Nut Snacks	28g	170	15	1	0	0	115	6
Bugles Original Corn Snacks	30g	160	9	8	0	0	310	18
Cape Cod Potato Chips	28g	150	8	0.5	0	0	110	17
Cape Cod Robust Russet Potato Chips	28g	150	8	0.5	0	0	150	16
Cape Cod Sea Salt & Vinegar Potato Chips	28g	150	8	0.5	0	0	130	17
Carr's Cracked Pepper Water Crackers	17g	70	1	0	0	0	100	13
Carr's Water Crackers	17g	70	1.5	0.5	0	0	100	13
Carr's Whole Wheat Snack Crackers	17g	80	3.5	1.5	0	0	100	11
Cheetos 100 Calorie Packs	18g	100	6	1.5	0	5	200	9
Cheetos Cheddar & Jalapeno Cheese Snacks	1 oz	170	11	1.5	0	5	250	15
Cheetos Cheese Snacks	28g	160	10	2	0	5	290	15
Cheetos Flamin' Hot Cheese Snacks	28g	170	11	1.5	0	5	250	15
Cheetos Natural White Cheddar Cheese Snacks	28g	150	9	1.5	0	0	290	16
Cheetos Go-Sack Cheese Snacks	28g	160	10	2	0	5	290	15
Clif Chocolate Chip Energy Bars	68g	240	5	1.5	0	0	140	44
Combos Cheddar Cheese Pretzels	28g	130	4.5	3	0	0	440	19

Snacks

Snacks	Serving	Calories	Total fat (gm)	Saturated fat (gm)	Trans fats (gm)	Cholesterol (mg)	Sodium (mg)	Carbs (gm)
Crunch N' Munch Butter Toffee & Peanut Popcorn	31g	140	5	1.5	0	5	160	23
Dare Breton Original Snack Crackers	13g	60	2.5	1.5	0	0	110	8
David All Natural Pumpkin Seeds	30g	160	12	2.5	0	0	10	4
David Original Sunflower Seeds	30g	190	15	1.5	0	0	135	5
Dole Dark Raisins	40g	120	0	0	0	0	0	32
Doritos 100 Calorie Packs	19g	100	6	1	0	0	140	12
Doritos Blazin' Buffalo & Ranch Tortilla Chips	28g	140	7	1	0	0	250	18
Doritos Cool Ranch Tortilla Chips	28g	150	8	1	0	0	180	18
Doritos Cooler Ranch Tortilla Chips	28g	140	7	1	0	0	180	18
Doritos Nacho Cheese Tortilla Chips	170g	150	8	1.5	0	0	180	17
Doritos Pizza Cravers & Ranch Tortilla Chips	28g	150	8	1.5	0	0	230	16
Doritos Spicy Nacho Tortilla Chips	28g	140	7	1	0	0	210	18
Doritos Spicy Sweet Chili Tortilla Chips	28g	140	7	1	0	0	270	18
Doritos Zesty Taco & Chipotle Ranch Tortilla Chips	28g	150	8	1	0	0	220	18
Eat Smart Original Vegetable Crisps	30g	140	7	0.5	0	0	290	18
El Ranchero Original Tortilla Chips	12	140	6	0	0	0	10	19
Emerald Almond Snack Nuts	¼ cup	160	14	1	0	0	150	6
Emerald Cashew Snack Nuts	¼ cup	160	14	2.5	0	0	85	9
Emerald Dark Chocolate Almond Snacks	¼ cup	150	13	1	0	0	25	6
Emerald Deluxe Mixed Nuts	¼ cup	170	16	2	0	0	75	5
Frito-Lay Original Sunflower Seeds	30g	190	16	1.5	0	0	360	5
Frito-Lay Go Snacks Nacho Cheese Tortilla Chips	28g	150	8	1.5	0	0	180	17
Fritos Barbecue Corn Chips	28g	150	10	1.5	0	0	290	16
Fritos Chili Cheese Corn Chips	28g	160	10	1.5	0	0	260	15
Fritos Flavor Twists Honey Barbecue Corn Snacks	28g	150	9	1.5	0	0	180	16
Fritos Honey Barbecue Corn Chips	28g	150	9	1.5	0	0	180	16
Fritos Original Corn Chips	28g	160	10	1.5	0	0	170	15
Fritos Scoops Original Corn Chips	28g	160	10	1.5	0	0	110	16
Funyuns Onion Rings	28g	140	7	1	0	0	240	18
Funyuns Onion Snacks	28g	140	7	1	0	0	240	18
Funyuns Go Sack Onion Salted Snacks	21g	110	5	0.5	0	0	180	14
Garden of Eatin' Blue Chips Original Tortilla Chips	28g	140	7	0.5	0	0	60	18
Gardetto's Snak-Ens Original Snack Mix	30g	150	6	1	1	0	270	20
General Mills Cheddar Chex Mix	27g	120	3.5	0.5	0	0	210	20
General Mills Cheerios Snack Mix	31g	120	3.5	0.5	0	0	330	21

Snacks

Snacks	Serving	Calories	Total fat (gm)	Saturated fat (gm)	Trans fats (gm)	Cholesterol (mg)	Sodium (mg)	Carbs (gm)
General Mills Chocolate Chex Mix	35g	140	3	0	0	0	135	26
General Mills Chocolate Turtle Chex Mix	28g	130	4.5	2	0	5	130	20
General Mills Fiber One Oat, Strawberry & Almond Snack Bars	40g	140	3	0.5	0	0	90	29
General Mills Fiber One Oats & Apple Streusel Snack Bars	40g	130	2	0.5	0	0	120	31
General Mills Fiber One Oats & Caramel Snack Bars	40g	140	3.5	1.5	0	0	105	30
General Mills Fiber One Oats & Chocolate Snack Bars	40g	140	4	1.5	0	0	90	29
General Mills Fiber One Oats & Peanut Butter Snack Bars	40g	150	4.5	2	0	0	105	28
General Mills Honey Nut Chex Mix	30g	130	4	0.5	0	0	280	23
General Mills Party Blend Chex Mix	30g	140	6	1	0.5	0	390	20
General Mills Peanut Lovers Chex Mix	30g	140	5	1	0	0	340	19
General Mills Traditional Chex Mix	30g	130	4	0.5	0	0	380	22
General Mills Turtle Chex Mix	35g	130	3.5	1	0	0	160	26
Herr's Original Tortillas Chip Dippers	1 oz	140	6	1.5	0	0	90	18
Herr's Potato Chips	1 oz	140	8	2.5	0	0	180	16
Herr's Rippled Potato Chips	1 oz	150	10	3	0	0	310	14
Herr's Sour Cream & Onion Potato Chips	1 oz	150	10	3	0	0	310	14
Jack Link's Original Beef Jerky	28g	80	1	0	0	20	590	3
Jiffy Pop Butter Kernel Popcorn	34g	140	7	1	3	0	220	19
Jolly Time Blast-O-Butter Ultimate Theater Style Microwave Popcorn	35g	150	12	3	4	0	340	19
Kashi TLC 7 Grain Snack Crackers	30g	130	3	0	0	0	160	22
Kashi TLC Cherry Dark Chocolate Granola Bars	35g	120	2	0.5	0	0	75	24
Kashi TLC Honey Almond Flax Granola Bars	35g	140	5	0.5	0	0	115	19
Kashi TLC Peanut Butter Granola Bars	35g	140	5	0.5	0	0	90	19
Kashi TLC Pumpkin Spice Flax Granola Bars	40g	180	6	0.5	0	0	150	26
Kashi TLC Trail Mix Granola Bars	35g	140	5	0.5	0	0	105	20
Keebler Club Buttery Garlic Snack Crackers	14g	70	3	0.5	0	0	150	9
Keebler Club Cheddar Cheese Sandwich Crackers	36g	190	10	2.5	0	0	360	23
Keebler Club Multigrain Snack Crackers	14g	70	3	0	0	0	130	9
Keebler Club Original Snack Crackers	16g	70	2	0	0	0	180	12
Keebler Peanut Butter Sandwich Crackers	39g	200	10	1.5	0	0	400	23
Keebler Toasted Butter Crisp Snack Crackers	16g	80	3.5	1	0	0	150	10
Keebler Toasted Onion Snack Crackers	16g	80	3.5	1	0	0	160	11
Keebler Toasted Sesame Snack Crackers	16g	80	3.5	1	0	0	140	10

Snacks

	Serving	Calories	Total fat (gm)	Saturated fat (gm)	Trans fats (gm)	Cholesterol (mg)	Sodium (mg)	Carbs (gm)
Keebler Toasted Wheat Snack Crackers	16g	80	3.5	0.5	0	0	150	10
Keebler Townhouse Bistro Multigrain Snack Crackers	16g	80	3	0.5	0	0	130	11
Keebler Townhouse Buttery Snack Crackers	15g	60	1.5	0.5	0	0	160	11
Keebler Townhouse Flipsides Cheddar Pretzels	15g	70	3.5	0.5	0	0	200	9
Keebler Townhouse Flipsides Original Pretzels	15g	70	3.5	0.5	0	0	200	10
Keebler Townhouse Regular Snack Crackers	16g	80	4.5	1	0	0	140	9
Keebler Townhouse Toppers Original Snack Crackers	14g	70	3	0.5	0	0	135	9
Keebler Townhouse Toppers Garlic & Herb Snack Crackers	14g	70	3	0.5	0	0	135	10
Keebler Townhouse Wheat Snack Crackers	16g	80	4	0.5	0	0	170	10
Keebler Wheatables Toasted Honey Wheat Snack Crackers	30g	140	6	1.5	0	0	310	20
Keebler Zesta Original Saltine Crackers	15g	60	1.5	0	0	0	200	11
Keebler Grahams Original Graham Crackers	29g	130	3.5	1	0	0	160	22
Kellogg's All Bran Multigrain Snack Crackers	30g	130	6	1	0	0	270	19
Kellogg's All Bran Garlic & Herb Snack Crackers	30g	120	6	1	0	0	330	19
Kellogg's Disney Pixar Finding Nemo Fruit Snacks	25g	80	0	0	0	0	5	19
Kellogg's Disney Princess Fruit Snacks	25g	80	0	0	0	0	5	19
Kellogg's Fiber Plus Chocolate Chip Granola Bars	36g	120	4	2	0	0	55	26
Kellogg's Fiber Plus Dark Chocolate Almond Granola Bars	36g	130	5	2.5	0	0	50	24
Kellogg's Rice Krispies Treats	22g	90	2.5	1	0	0	105	17
Kellogg's Special K Chocolatey Drizzle Cereal Bars	22g	90	1.5	1	0	0	105	17
Kellogg's Special K Peaches & Berries Cereal Bars	23g	90	2	1	0	0	85	18
Kellogg's Special K Strawberry Cereal Bars	23g	90	1.5	1	0	0	95	18
Kellogg's Special K Vanilla Crisp Cereal Bars	22g	90	1.5	1	0	0	100	17
Kellogg's Sponge Bob Square Pants Fruit Snacks	25g	80	0	0	0	0	5	19
Kettle Potato Chips	28g	150	9	1	0	0	105	16
Kettle Salt & Fresh Green Pepper Potato Chips	28g	150	9	1	0	0	180	16
Kettle Sea Salt & Vinegar Potato Chips	28g	150	9	1	0	0	190	16
Kraft Handi-Snacks Premium Cheese Breadsticks with Spread	31g	110	4.5	1	0	5	350	14

Snacks

Snacks	Serving	Calories	Total fat (gm)	Saturated fat (gm)	Trans fats (gm)	Cholesterol (mg)	Sodium (mg)	Carbs (gm)
Kraft Macaroni & Cheese Cheddar Snack Crackers	30g	150	7	2	0	5	280	18
Kraft South Beach Diet High Protein Cereal Bars	35g	140	5	3.5	0	0	150	15
Lance Assorted Sandwich Crackers	43g	220	11	2	0	5	430	23
Lay's Barbecue Potato Chips	28g	150	10	1	0	0	200	15
Lay's Cheddar & Sour Cream Potato Chips	28g	160	10	1	0	5	230	15
Lay's Classic Potato Chips	28g	150	10	1	0	0	180	15
Lay's Kettle Cooked Barbecue Potato Chips	28g	150	10	1	0	0	200	15
Lay's Kettle Cooked Jalapeno Potato Chips	1 oz	140	8	1	0	0	170	16
Lay's Kettle Cooked Mesquite Barbecue Potato Chips	28g	140	8	1	0	0	210	16
Lay's Kettle Cooked Original Potato Chips	28g	150	8	1	0	0	110	18
Lay's Kettle Cooked Salt & Vinegar Potato Chips	1 oz	140	7	1	0	0	260	17
Lay's Light Fat Free Potato Chips	28g	75	0	0	0	0	200	17
Lay's Natural Sea Salt Potato Chips	28g	150	10	1	0	0	150	15
Lay's Salt & Vinegar Potato Chips	28g	150	10	1	0	0	380	15
Lay's Sour Cream & Onion Potato Chips	28g	160	10	1	0	0	210	15
Lay's Stax Original Potato Crisps	28g	150	9	1	0	0	160	16
Mariani Whole Dried Cranberries	40g	130	0	0	0	0	0	35
Mission Original Tortilla Chips	28g	140	7	2	0	0	150	17
Munchies Cheese Fix Snack Mix	28g	140	7	1	0	0	250	18
Munchos Potato Crisps	28g	160	10	1.5	0	0	230	16
Nabisco 100 Calorie Packs Cheese Nips	21g	100	3	1	0	0	230	15
Nabisco 100 Calorie Packs Milk Chocolate Pretzels	22g	100	3.5	2	0	0	160	16
Nabisco 100 Calorie Packs Ritz Snack Mix	22g	100	3	0.5	0	0	210	16
Nabisco Cheese Nips Cheddar Snack Crackers	30g	150	6	1.5	0	0	340	19
Nabisco Flavor Originals Better Cheddars Snack Crackers	31g	160	8	1.5	0	5	360	18
Nabisco Flavor Originals Chicken in A Biscuit Snack Crackers	31g	160	8	1.5	0	0	300	19
Nabisco Flavor Originals Sociables Snack Crackers	14g	70	3.5	0.5	0	0	140	9
Nabisco Flavor Originals Vegetable Thins Snack Crackers	30g	150	7	2	0	0	320	19
Nabisco Honey Maid Cinnamon Graham Crackers	31g	130	2.5	0.5	0	0	170	25
Nabisco Honey Maid Honey Graham Crackers	31g	130	3	0.5	0	0	190	24
Nabisco Low Fat Honey Maid Cinnamon Graham Crackers	31g	120	1.5	0	0	0	180	26

Snacks

	Serving	Calories	Total fat (gm)	Saturated fat (gm)	Trans fats (gm)	Cholesterol (mg)	Sodium (mg)	Carbs (gm)
Nabisco Low Fat Honey Maid Honey Graham Crackers	31g	120	2	0	0	0	190	25
Nabisco Low Saturated Fat Honey Maid Honey Graham Crackers	31g	130	3	0.5	0	0	190	24
Nabisco Newtons Apple Cinnamon Fruit Crisps	28g	100	2	0	0	0	90	20
Nabisco Newtons Mixed Berry Fruit Crisps	28g	100	2	0	0	0	85	20
Nabisco Original Graham Crackers	31g	130	3	0.5	0	0	190	24
Nabisco Premium Low Sodium Saltine Crackers	15g	60	1.5	0	0	0	30	12
Nabisco Premium Multigrain Saltine Crackers	14g	60	1.5	0	0	0	170	10
Nabisco Premium Original Saltine Crackers	15g	70	2	0.5	0	0	150	11
Nabisco Premium Regular Saltine Crackers	16g	60	0	0	0	0	200	13
Nabisco Premium Soup & Oyster Crackers	15g	60	1.5	0	0	0	170	11
Nabisco Premium Unsalted Tops Saltine Crackers	15g	70	1.5	0	0	0	95	11
Nabisco Ritz Bits Cheese Sandwich Crackers	28g	150	8	3	0	0	240	16
Nabisco Ritz Bits Peanut Butter Sandwich Crackers	29g	140	8	1.5	0	0	240	16
Nabisco Ritz Cheese Sandwich Crackers	38g	200	12	3	0	5	440	21
Nabisco Ritz Fresh Stacks Snack Crackers	16g	80	4.5	1	0	0	135	10
Nabisco Ritz Honey Butter Snack Crackers	16g	80	4	1	0	0	70	10
Nabisco Ritz Peanut Butter Sandwich Crackers	39g	200	11	1.5	0	0	400	21
Nabisco Ritz Regular Snack Crackers	15g	70	2	0	0	0	160	11
Nabisco Ritz Roasted Vegetable Snack Crackers	16g	80	3.5	1	0	0	150	10
Nabisco Ritz Toasted Cheddar Chips	30g	130	6	1	0	0	290	19
Nabisco Ritz Toasted Original Chips	28g	130	4.5	0.5	0	0	290	21
Nabisco Ritz Toasted Sour Cream & Onion Chips	28g	130	6	1	0	0	270	19
Nabisco Ritz Toasted Garlic Mozzarella Chips	39g	200	10	1.5	2	0	410	23
Nabisco Ritz Whole Wheat Snack Crackers	15g	70	2.5	0.5	0	0	120	11
Nabisco Snowflake Ritz Snack Crackers	16g	80	4.5	1	0	0	150	10
Nabisco Triscuit Cracked Pepper & Olive Oil Snack Crackers	28g	120	4	1	0	0	140	20
Nabisco Triscuit Fire Roasted Tomato & Olive Oil Snack Crackers	28g	120	4	1	0	0	150	20
Nabisco Triscuit Original Snack Crackers	28g	120	4.5	1	0	0	180	19
Nabisco Triscuit Original Thin Crisps	30g	130	5	1	0	0	180	21
Nabisco Triscuit Parmesan Garlic Thin Crisps	31g	140	5	1	0	0	180	22

Snacks

Snacks	Serving	Calories	Total fat (gm)	Saturated fat (gm)	Trans fats (gm)	Cholesterol (mg)	Sodium (mg)	Carbs (gm)
Nabisco Triscuit Reduced Fat Wheat Snack Crackers	29g	120	3	0.5	0	0	160	21
Nabisco Triscuit Roasted Garlic Snack Crackers	28g	120	4.5	1	0	0	140	20
Nabisco Triscuit Rosemary & Olive Oil Snack Crackers	28g	120	4	1	0	0	135	20
Nabisco Triscuit Rosemary & Olive Oil Wheat Snack Crackers	28g	120	4	0.5	0	0	135	20
Nabisco Triscuit Rye Snack Crackers	28g	120	4.5	1	0	0	150	19
Nabisco Triscuit Thin Crisps Quattro Formaggio Snack Crackers	31g	140	4.5	1	0	0	160	22
Nabisco Triscuit Garden Herb Snack Crackers	28g	120	4	1	0	0	125	20
Nabisco Wheat Thins Country French Onion Snack Crackers	31g	140	4	0.5	0	0	290	23
Nabisco Wheat Thins Cream Cheese & Chive Snack Crackers	29g	140	5	1	0	0	260	22
Nabisco Wheat Thins Fiber Selects 5 Grain Snack Crackers	30g	120	4.5	0.5	0	0	260	22
Nabisco Wheat Thins Fiber Selects Garden Vegetable Snack Crackers	30g	120	4	0.5	0	0	260	22
Nabisco Wheat Thins Multigrain Snack Crackers	31g	140	4.5	1	0	0	230	22
Nabisco Wheat Thins Original Snack Crackers	29g	130	4	0.5	0	0	260	21
Nabisco Wheat Thins Parmesan Basil Snack Crackers	30g	140	5	1	0	0	290	21
Nabisco Wheat Thins Ranch Snack Crackers	29g	140	6	1	0	0	230	19
Nabisco Wheat Thins Sun Dried Tomato & Basil Snack Crackers	30g	140	6	1	0	0	240	20
Nabisco Wheat Thins Toasted Multigrain Chips	28g	120	4	0.5	0	0	240	20
Nabisco Wheat Thins Toasted Parmesan Herb Chips	28g	130	5	1	0	0	270	19
Nabisco Wheat Thins Toasted Veggie Chips	30g	120	4	0.5	0	0	290	20
Nabisco Wheat Thins Whole Grain Snack Crackers	31g	140	6	1	0	0	290	21
Nature Valley Fruit & Nut Trail Mix Bars	35g	140	4	0.5	0	0	100	25
Nature Valley Maple Brown Sugar Granola Bars	42g	180	6	0.5	0	0	160	29
Nature Valley Oats & Honey Granola Bars	42g	180	6	0.5	0	0	160	29
Nature Valley Peanut Butter Granola Bars	42g	180	7	1	0	0	190	30
Nature Valley Pecan Crunch Granola Bars	42g	190	7	1	0	0	170	29
Nature Valley Roasted Almond Granola Bars	42g	190	7	1	0	0	180	28

Snacks	Serving	Calories	Total fat (gm)	Saturated fat (gm)	Trans fats (gm)	Cholesterol (mg)	Sodium (mg)	Carbs (gm)
Nature Valley Roasted Nut Crunch Granola Bars	35g	190	13	1.5	0	0	180	13
Nature Valley Sweet & Salty Nut Cashew Granola Bars	35g	160	7	2.5	0	0	150	22
Nature Valley Sweet & Salty Nut Peanut Granola Bars	35g	170	9	2.5	0	0	150	19
Nature Valley Sweet & Salty Nut Roasted Mixed Nut Granola Bars	35g	160	8	2.5	0	0	150	21
New York Style Original Bagel Crisps	28g	130	6	2.5	0	0	70	18
New York Style Roasted Garlic Bagel Crisps	28g	130	6	2.5	0	0	470	17
New York Style Sea Salt Bagel Crisps	28g	130	6	2.5	0	0	360	18
Ocean Spray Cherry Craisins	40g	130	0	0	0	0	0	33
Ocean Spray Original Craisins	40g	130	0	0	0	0	0	33
Oh Boy! Oberto Original Beefsteak Jerky	28g	70	1	0	0	10	450	7
On The Border Mexican Grill & Cantina Tortilla Chips	28g	140	7	1	0	0	80	19
Orville Redenbacher 50% Less Fat Butter Microwave Popcorn	31g	120	5	2.5	0	0	190	19
Orville Redenbacher Butter Microwave Popcorn	35g	170	12	6	0	0	260	17
Orville Redenbacher Butter Popcorn Popping Oil	14ml	120	14	2	0	0	0	0
Orville Redenbacher No Trans Fat Butter Microwave Popcorn	35g	170	12	6	0	0	260	17
Orville Redenbacher No Trans Fat Microwave Kettle Corn	34g	170	13	7	0	5	130	16
Orville Redenbacher No Trans Fat Movie Theater Butter Microwave Popcorn	43g	210	15	7	0	0	300	20
Orville Redenbacher No Trans Fat Ultimate Butter Microwave Popcorn	34g	170	12	6	0	0	380	16
Orville Redenbacher Original Kernel Popcorn	40g	120	1.5	0	0	0	0	29
Orville Redenbacher Smart Pop 94% Fat Free Butter Microwave Popcorn	37g	120	2	0.5	0	0	240	25
Orville Redenbacher Smart Pop 94% Fat Free Microwave Kettle Corn	42g	140	2	1	0	0	230	29
Orville Redenbacher Tender White Microwave Popcorn	33g	170	12	6	0	0	250	15
Pepperidge Farm Cheddar Goldfish Crackers	30g	140	5	1	0	5	250	20
Pepperidge Farm Colors Goldfish Crackers	30g	140	5	1	0	5	260	20
Pepperidge Farm Entertaining Quartet Crackers	15g	70	2.5	0.5	0	5	100	10
Pepperidge Farm Flavor Blasted Xplosive Pizza Goldfish Crackers	30g	140	6	0.5	0	0	280	19
Pepperidge Farm Flavor Blasted Xtra Cheddar Goldfish Crackers	30g	140	6	1	0	5	310	18

Snacks

Snacks	Serving	Calories	Total fat (gm)	Saturated fat (gm)	Trans fats (gm)	Cholesterol (mg)	Sodium (mg)	Carbs (gm)
Pepperidge Farm Parmesan Cheese Goldfish Crackers	30g	130	4	1	0	0	280	20
Pepperidge Farm Pizza Goldfish Crackers	30g	140	5	1	0	0	230	20
Pepperidge Farm Pretzel Thins	28g	110	0	0	0	0	390	21
Pepperidge Farm Pretzel Goldfish Crackers	30g	130	2.5	0.5	0	0	430	24
Pepperidge Farm Whole Grain Goldfish Crackers	30g	140	5	1	0	5	250	19
Planters Cashew Snack Nuts	28g	160	13	2.5	0	0	115	9
Planters Cocktail Peanut Snacks	28g	170	14	2	0	0	115	5
Planters Deluxe Mixed Nuts	28g	170	15	2	0	0	105	7
Planters Honey Peanuts	28g	160	12	1.5	0	0	115	8
Planters Mixed Nuts & Peanuts	125g	70	3	0.5	0	0	460	9
Planters No Shell Sunflower Kernals	31g	180	15	1.5	0	0	260	6
Planters NUTrition Almonds	28g	160	15	1	0	0	40	5
Planters NUTrition Cashew, Almond & Macadamia Nuts	28g	170	15	2	0	0	50	7
Planters NUTrition Chocolate Nut Mix	33g	160	10	2.5	0	0	20	16
Planters NUTrition Fruit & Nut Snacks	32g	150	8	1	0	0	45	17
Planters NUTrition Mixed Nut Snacks	28g	170	16	1.5	0	0	45	5
Planters Peanuts	28g	170	14	2	0	0	0	5
Planters Pistachio & Mixed Nut Snacks	28g	160	13	1.5	0	0	80	7
Planters Redskin Spanish Peanuts	28g	180	15	2.5	0	0	115	5
Planters Select Cashew, Almond & Pecan Snack Nuts	28g	170	15	2	0	0	95	7
Pop Secret 100 Calorie Pop Butter Microwave Popcorn	31g	110	3.5	1.5	0	0	300	20
Pop Secret 94% Fat Free Butter Microwave Popcorn	39g	140	2	1	0	0	420	26
Pop Secret Butter Microwave Popcorn	36g	180	11	2.5	5	0	330	17
Pop Secret Extra Butter Microwave Popcorn	36g	190	12	2	5	0	300	17
Pop Secret Movie Theater Butter Microwave Popcorn	36g	180	12	2.5	5	0	300	18
Pop Secret Salted Homestyle Butter Microwave Popcorn	36g	180	11	1.5	5	0	410	18
Popcorn Indiana Trans Fat Free Kettle Corn	28g	130	5	0	0	0	130	21
Pringles Barbecue Potato Crisps	28g	150	10	3	0	0	160	14
Pringles Cheddar Cheese Potato Crisps	28g	150	11	3	0	0	180	14
Pringles Fat Free Original Potato Crisps	28g	70	0	0	0	0	160	15
Pringles Fat Free Sour Cream & Onion Potato Crisps	28g	70	0	0	0	0	190	15
Pringles Original Potato Crisps	184g	140	10	3	0	0	150	12
Pringles Original Reduced Fat Potato Crisps	28g	140	8	2	0	0	135	17

Snacks	Serving	Calories	Total fat (gm)	Saturated fat (gm)	Trans fats (gm)	Cholesterol (mg)	Sodium (mg)	Carbs (gm)
Pringles Pizza-Licious Potato Crisps	28g	150	10	3	0	0	190	14
Pringles Salt & Vinegar Potato Crisps	28g	150	10	3	0	0	220	14
Pringles Sour Cream & Onion Potato Crisps	28g	150	10	3	0	0	180	14
Pringles Stix Honey Butter Crackers	19g	90	3.5	1.5	0	0	150	12
Pringles Stix Pizza Crackers	19g	90	4	2	0	0	140	11
Pringles Super Stack Original Potato Crisps	28g	150	9	2.5	0	0	160	15
Pringles Super Stack Sour Cream & Onion Potato Crisps	28g	150	9	2.5	0	0	170	15
Quaker Apple Cinnamon Rice Cakes	13g	50	0	0	0	0	0	11
Quaker Caramel Corn Rice Cakes	13g	50	0	0	0	0	30	11
Quaker Chewy 90 Calories Chocolate Granola Bars	24g	90	2	0.5	0	0	80	19
Quaker Chewy 90 Calories Dark Chocolate & Cherry Granola Bars	24g	90	2	0.5	0	0	75	19
Quaker Chewy 90 Calories Oatmeal Raisin Granola Bars	24g	90	1.5	0	0	0	80	19
Quaker Chewy Chocolate Chip Granola Bars	24g	100	3.5	1	0	0	75	17
Quaker Chewy Dipps Chocolate Chip Granola Bars	31g	140	5	2.5	0	0	80	22
Quaker Chewy Dipps Peanut Butter Granola Bars	30g	150	7	2.5	0.5	0	100	19
Quaker Chewy Peanut Butter & Chocolate Chip Granola Bars	24g	100	3	1	0	0	75	17
Quaker Chewy Peanut Butter & Chocolate Hi Protein Granola Bars	28g	110	3	1	0	0	140	18
Quaker Chewy S'More Granola Bars	24g	100	2	0.5	0	0	80	19
Quaker Mini Delights Caramel Drizzle Bitesize Rice Cakes	20g	90	3.5	3	0	0	95	14
Quaker Mini Delights Chocolatey Drizzle Bitesize Rice Cakes	20g	90	3.5	3.5	0	0	85	14
Quaker Quakes Flavored Mini Rice Snacks	16g	60	0	0	0	0	50	15
Quaker Simple Harvest Dark Chocolate Granola Bars	35g	150	4.5	1.5	0	0	95	26
Quaker White Cheddar Rice Cakes	11g	45	0.5	0	0	0	105	8
Red Oval Farms Stoned Wheat Thins	14g	60	1.5	0	0	0	210	10
Robert's American Gourmet Pirate's Booty	28g	130	5	1	0	0	150	18
Rold Gold Cheddar Cheese Pretzels	28g	110	1	0	0	0	370	22
Rold Gold Fat Free Pretzels	28g	100	0	0	0	0	420	23
Rold Gold Honey Mustard Pretzels	28g	110	1	0	0	0	430	23
Rold Gold Honey Wheat Pretzels	28g	110	1	0	0	0	230	23
Rold Gold Pretzels	28g	110	1	0	0	0	560	23
Ruffles Cheddar & Sour Cream Potato Chips	28g	160	11	1.5	0	0	230	14

Snacks

Snacks	Serving	Calories	Total fat (gm)	Saturated fat (gm)	Trans fats (gm)	Cholesterol (mg.)	Sodium (mg.)	Carbs (nm)
Ruffles Cheddar Potato Chips	28g	160	10	1.5	0	0	260	15
Ruffles Fat Free Potato Chips	28g	70	0	0	0	0	190	17
Ruffles Natural Potato Chips	28g	140	7	0.5	0	0	160	17
Ruffles Original Potato Chips	28g	160	10	1	0	0	160	14
Ruffles Reduced Fat Potato Chips	28g	140	7	1	0	0	180	18
Ruffles Sour Cream & Onion Potato Chips	28g	160	11	1.5	0	0	190	14
S & W Pik-Nik Original Potato Snacks	28g	160	10	3	5	0	100	15
Santitas Original Tortilla Chips	28g	130	6	1	0	0	110	19
Slim Jim Chicken & Beef Jerky	28g	150	13	5	1	35	420	2
Slim Jim Original Beef Jerky	32g	170	14	6	1	20	490	2
Smartfood Trans Fat Free White Cheddar Cheese Popcorn	18g	100	6	1.5	0	5	200	9
Smartfood White Cheddar Cheese Popcorn	28g	160	10	2	0	5	290	14
Snyder's of Hanover Butter Pretzels	30g	120	1	0	0	0	270	25
Snyder's of Hanover Cheddar Cheese Pretzels	28g	150	8	4	0	5	200	16
Snyder's of Hanover Cheddar Sourdough Pretzels	28g	130	6	3.5	0	0	260	18
Snyder's of Hanover Fat Free Pretzels	30g	110	0	0	0	0	75	25
Snyder's of Hanover Fat Free Sourdough Pretzels	28g	100	0	0	0	0	240	22
Snyder's of Hanover Hot Buffalo Wing Pretzels	28g	140	7	3	0	0	380	17
Snyder's of Hanover Low Fat Pretzels	30g	120	1	0	0	0	390	25
Snyder's of Hanover Olde Tyme Pretzels	30g	120	1	0	0	0	120	24
Snyder's of Hanover Original Tortilla Chips	28g	140	4.5	0	0	0	135	23
Snyder's of Hanover Peanut Butter Pretzels	28g	140	7	2	0	0	140	16
Snyder's of Hanover Regular Pretzels	30g	110	1	0	0	0	300	23
Snyder's of Hanover Sourdough Honey Mustard & Onion Pretzels	30g	130	3	1.5	0	0	95	23
Stacy's Cinnamon Sugar Pita Chips	28g	140	5	0.5	0	0	115	20
Stacy's Multigrain Pita Chips	28g	140	5	0.5	0	0	270	19
Stacy's Parmesan, Garlic & Herb Pita Chips	28g	140	5	0.5	0	0	200	19
Stacy's Simply Naked Pita Chips	28g	130	5	0.5	0	0	270	19
Sunbelt Chocolate Chip Granola Bars	35g	170	7	4	0	0	60	24
Sunbelt Fudge Dipped Chocolate Chip Granola Bars	43g	210	10	6	0	0	70	29
Sunbelt Oats & Honey Granola Bars	28g	130	5	3	0	0	65	19
Sunchips Flavored Multigrain Chips	28g	140	6	1	0	0	130	18
Sunchips Original Multigrain Chips	28g	140	6	1	0	0	120	18
Sunkist Pistachios	30g	170	14	1.5	0	0	160	8
Sun-Maid Cape Cod Dried Cranberries	40g	130	0	0	0	0	0	33

Snacks	Serving	Calories	Total fat (gm)	Saturated fat (gm)	Trans fats (gm)	Cholesterol (mg)	Sodium (mg)	Carbs (gm)
Sun-Maid Dark Chocolate Yogurt Raisins	43g	130	0	0	0	0	10	33
Sun-Maid Original Raisins	40g	130	0	0	0	0	10	31
Sun-Maid Vanilla Yogurt Raisins	30g	130	5	4	0	0	20	21
Sun-Maid Golden Raisins	40g	130	0	0	0	0	10	31
Sunshine Big Cheez-It Cheese Crackers	30g	160	8	2	0	0	250	18
Sunshine Cheez-It Assorted Party Mix	30g	120	4.5	1	0	0	290	21
Sunshine Cheez-It Cheddar Cheese Crackers	35g	180	9	2	0.5	0	300	21
Sunshine Cheez-It Cheddar Jack Crackers	30g	140	7	1	0	0	240	17
Sunshine Cheez-It Duoz Sharp Chedder & Parmesan Crackers	30g	150	8	2	0	0	260	18
Sunshine Cheez-It Hot & Spicy Crackers	30g	150	8	2	0	0	300	18
Sunshine Cheez-It White Cheddar Crackers	30g	150	8	2.5	0	0	280	18
Sunshine Krispy Saltine Crackers	15g	60	1.5	0	0	0	200	11
Sunshine Right Bites Cheez-It Cheese Crackers	22g	100	3	1	0	0	230	15
Sunsweet Pitted Prunes	40g	100	0	0	0	0	5	24
Terra Original Vegetable Chips	28g	150	9	1	0	0	50	16
The Snack Factory Everything Pretzel Crisps	28g	110	0.5	0	0	0	170	23
The Snack Factory Original Pretzel Crisps	28g	110	0	0	0	0	330	23
Tostitos Light Tortilla Chips	28g	90	1	0	0	0	105	20
Tostitos Multigrain Tortilla Chips	28g	150	8	1	0	0	135	18
Tostitos Natural Original Tortilla Chips	28g	140	6	0.5	0	0	80	19
Tostitos Original Tortilla Chips	28g	140	8	1	0	0	110	18
Tostitos Scoops Hint of Jalapeno Tortilla Chips	28g	140	7	1	0	0	135	19
Tostitos Scoops Original Tortilla Chips	28g	140	7	1	0	0	120	18
Utz Barbecue Potato Chips	28g	150	10	2.5	0	0	240	14
Utz Sour Cream & Onion Potato Chips	28g	160	10	3	0	0	140	14
Utz Sourdough Pretzels	28g	110	1	0	0	0	470	21
Wasa Multigrain Crisps	14g	45	0	0	0	0	80	10
Wavy Lay's Hickory Barbecue Potato Chips	28g	150	10	1	0	0	210	16
Wavy Lay's Original Potato Chips	28g	150	10	1	0	0	180	15
Wavy Lay's Ranch Potato Chips	28g	150	10	1.5	0	0	200	16
Wise Barbecue Potato Chips	28g	150	10	3	0	0	210	14
Wise Cheez Doodles Cheese Snacks	28g	150	8	2	0	0	320	17
Wise Honey Barbecue Potato Chips	28g	150	10	2.5	0	0	190	15
Wise Regular Potato Chips	28g	150	10	3	0	0	160	14

Grocery Index

A

B

Grocery Index

Grocery Index

Grocery Index

Grocery Index

L

M

N

Grocery Index

S

Grocery Index

Grocery Index

NOTES:

NOTES:

Why not share The Stop & Go Grocery Guide or Fast Food Guide with all your friends and family?

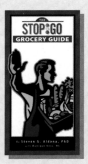

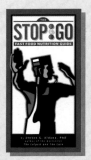

Grocery Guide   **Fast Food Guide**

They make perfect gifts for those you really care about.

- Give a copy of the guides for Mother's Day or Father's Day to show your parents you really care about them and want them to be around for a long time.
- If you are a physician, why not give a copy of each to your patients?
- If you are an employer, why not show your employees you really value them by giving each of them a copy.

Order more than one copy and save!

Quantity	Your Cost Per Guide
1	6.95
2–9	4.95
10–99	3.95
100–999	2.95
1,000 +	Call

To order, go to www.welcoa.org or contact us at:

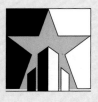

Wellness Council of America
9802 Nicholas Street, Suite 315
Omaha, NE 68114

Phone: (402) 827-3590
Fax: (402) 827-3594
Email: wellworkplace@welcoa.org

Are you ready to:

- Cut through the diet and health hype and learn the facts?
- Reach a healthy weight and maintain it for life?
- Extend your life by 10–20 years?
- Prevent the diseases your physician can only treat?
- Understand how your daily choices directly affect your health?

If you are really ready to improve your health, then Dr. Aldana's best-selling book, *The Culprit and The Cure,* is the book for you. As one of the nation's leading experts on healthy living, Dr. Aldana will help you learn how your body will change when you enjoy good nutrition and regular physical activity. You will see how these changes can help prevent, arrest, and even reverse many chronic diseases. You'll get realistic tips, goals, and ideas on how to eat right and exercise, and you'll begin to enjoy a long, high quality life. Your own health—and life—transformation begins the moment you open its pages.

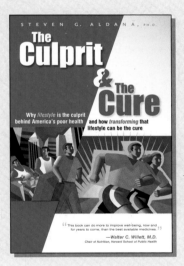

The Culprit and The Cure by Steven Aldana, PhD

Wellness Council of America
$9.95 ($2.95 for 2+ copies)

Read the first chapter right now at **www.welcoa.org**.

Dr. Steven Aldana is a former professor of Lifestyle Medicine in the Department of Exercise Sciences at Brigham Young University in Provo, Utah, and he is an adjunct faculty member of the University of Illinois School of Medicine. Currently, Dr. Aldana is the CEO of www.WellSteps.com. He has spent his career researching and teaching about the impact of lifestyle on disease and quality of life.

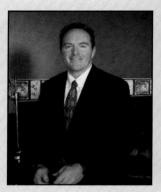

He has published over 60 research articles and has written five books on the connections between healthy living and disease prevention. He is a regular consultant to the Centers for Disease Control and Prevention, the National Institutes of Health, and the California Department of Health Services. In the past few years he has given over 80 invited lectures and keynote speeches around the United States. He has received numerous state, private, and federal grants to research how the adoption of healthy behaviors can prevent, arrest, and even reverse many common chronic diseases such as cardiovascular disease, diabetes, and cancer.

As one who practices what he preaches, Dr. Aldana is passionate about educating people about the tremendous impact lifestyle has on disease and is devoted to helping individuals adopt and maintain healthy lifestyles. As a nationally recognized expert on healthy living, he is a highly sought after speaker and advisor. He lives in the heart of the Rocky Mountains with his wife and children. When he is not working in his garden he can often be found playing flag football, mountain biking, or running.